Ema

Healed

BY THE MIRACLE HAND OF GOD

A Must read!

Book Layout © 2016 BookDesignTemplates.com

Healed by the Miracle hand of God/ Margaret Ema. -- 1st ed.
SBN-13: 978-1539845010
ISBN-10: 153984501X

Dedication

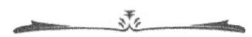

I dedicate this Book to you my precious friend!
This is an Epistle written especially to you

The concept of faith

When asked to describe faith, Dr Yonggi Cho answered with a question. He asked "if you throw an egg at a rock, which one will break? And the response was obvious. The egg should break of course. But he answered and said "wrong, it is the rock that will break instead of the egg" this is faith. The power to accomplish the impossible. He concluded by saying "always expect a miracle, expect God to do a miracle for you" believe God today!

Excerpt

"The scripture says that "how God anointed Jesus Christ of Nazareth with the Holy Ghost and with Power who went about doing good and healing all that were oppressed of the devil for God was with Him" Acts 10: 38.

That statement shows God in active partnership with His Son Jesus by His spirit to heal and deliver those oppressed of the devil, then what sense would it make for Him to go back to the devil to borrow his tools to afflict his children when they do wrong and sometimes do nothing at all just to teach them a lesson as some allude to"

"So, you see that it means a lot to God that you and I be healed and delivered so that we can bring the same blessing to many. God can then spread the Blessing through us to the rest of mankind. Whatever you are desiring from God today, see the bigger picture. Let God show you how much of a blessing it would be for you to be healed than for that condition to prolong in your life. Think about this, if you were God, what would you rather have, if you had the ability to do for your children what they desire, which one would you do? Which one will be a greater witness to your faithfulness and kindness? Which one will attract many to you? What would you rather do?"

Contents

PREFACE

Jesus the Healer is speaking to you through the pages of this epistle. Let the words of this book bring faith in your heart and renew in you the ability to simply take God at His word.

Mary and Martha told Jesus that the situation with their brother had passed the point of no return, because he was already dead and buried and corruption had set in. But Jesus knew better that faith in God can reverse any situation. Jesus answered Martha and said, "If you believe, you shall see the Glory or power of God" now my friend this is the key right there – the key to unlocking the supernatural power of God to work for us is our ability to simply believe God and take Him at His Word!

Supernatural supply: I walked into my children's bedroom many years ago and there was so much I desired in my heart to do in that room to make them more comfortable, but each time I thought of it, the spirit of lack and want rose up in my heart and I began to think of how I will ever have the money to do those things and that day as I thought the same way that I have always done for years, I heard the Holy Spirit say within me "why don't you believe that God will give you what you want"

I was startled because it never occurred to me that my situation was prolonged because of unbelief. I am full of the Word [notice that I said that I was full of the Word] but my problem was that each time I had a need or desire I began to try and figure out how it would happen. The facts on ground would amplify the impossibility and I would become overwhelmed.

At that point, my faith became unprogressive so I continued to remain in lack and want.

Unbelief and doubt are spirits and they are very subtle, they creep in unnoticed and produce fear and fear is the opposite of faith. Fear lets the devil work his plan in a person's life, fear means that God cannot be trusted and that the enemy is more powerful.

Fear magnifies the ability of the enemy or your situation. Fear makes that situation or condition become your god and shuts down your faith and disconnects you from the flow of God's Grace, power and ability, it keeps God out and so that situation prolongs and at the end it will accomplish the plan of the enemy.

While faith opens the door for God to come in with all His resources to partner with you to accomplish your desire, He brings His own faith to force a change for you.

You wonder how this relates to healing. You see everything in the Kingdom of God works on the same principles of faith which is that "you believe with your heart and doubt not in your heart" and "believe you receive when you pray" – that is it.

Take God at His word believe Him and keep doubt out, don't try to figure out how it will happen, just settle in your heart that it is done and Jesus said, "**Go your way** [meaning - go about your business] and it will be done for you according to your faith" as you have believed – That is your God given ability to believe based on what God has said.

Abraham believe according to that which was spoken "so shall your seed be" and based on that promise of God alone, he did not stagger in the face of opposing circumstance, but was fully persuaded that what God had promised, he was also able to perform it.

God will do for you as you have believed! Think about that for a moment. The Lord bless you as you read!

1

Lord Stretch forth your Hands to heal

As a foundation, I want you to see the miracle hand of the Lord the healer stretched out eagerly to you today. The book is based on the cry of the Disciples when faced with severe persecution, they had one cry, they said; Lord, "stretch forth Your hand to heal; and that signs and wonders may be done by the name of thy holy child Jesus.

The Lord's immediate response is to us a confirmation of the mind of God concerning healing. "And when they had prayed, the place was shaken where they were assembled together; and they were all filled with the Holy Ghost, and they spoke the word of God with boldness" Acts 4: 30.

Let this become your focus as you read this book. Keep your eye and focus on the healing hand of God and His complete willingness to heal you now as you believe.

Healing always comes

I have taken comfort many times in that statement. A servant of God testified that at a meeting a parent had brought their child to him and that child was afflicted with a severe case of epilepsy if I can remember correctly what the condition was but I know that it was very serious. This minister prayed a prayer of faith and released his faith for healing and it looked as though nothing happened or things got worse because the child had a seizure right there as he was prayed for.

He said he walked away wondering if anything had happened and the Lord assured him that there is healing and there is recovery, but the bottom line is that "healing always comes" Sure enough he said he was in another meeting a few months later and a family approached him but he could not recognize them and the mother then introduced herself and told this minister that as they returned home from that other meeting where they had previously met this preacher, their child began to recover and has been well since.

I pray for you: As you read this book, this will be your case because you will begin to recover and come to be well completely in every area of your life. The same way that condition came so it must go from you now by the authority in the name of our Lord Jesus Christ. Amen!

Fear not, for you shall Live

You know the greatest and I believe the main weapon of the devil is fear. In the same way that faith opens the door for God to intervene for us, fear gives the devil access to kill steal and destroy. Fear really means that God cannot be trusted and that the devil is too powerful and that the condition cannot be reversed by simply believing God.

If the devil can get fear to take root in your heart he can accomplish anything. That is why we must keep supplying our spirit man with the word of God where faith comes from so that faith will be produced for us continually. When my body is attacked, the enemy will begin to suggest to me that it is this, or it is that. You know what ever the symptom maybe any affliction has the spirit of infirmity behind it. We know that Jesus took infirmities for us and bore our sicknesses and we believe it.

In suggesting what you could have by that symptom, the enemy is looking for access to gain entrance through fear and your mental accent. He is looking for your agreement so that he can manifest that thing that he is suggesting. He also does that by magnifying everything so that you begin to fear. You are only afraid because he will immediately make you see the possibility of that thing resulting in death. His mission is to kill steal and destroy. But we must understand that the scripture is very clear about how we stand were death is concerned. Every fear of man has its root in the fear of death. Think about that for a moment.

Jesus by becoming flesh and dying has delivered us from that. This really liberated me from any fear of death, I know that I can receive healing from every attack in my body and if it is an oppression of any kind, I can take my deliverance and walk away free. Let me share my liberty with you. The scripture says;

> Forasmuch then as the children are partakers of flesh and blood, he also himself likewise took part of the same; that through death he might destroy him that had the power of death, that is, the devil;
>
> 15 And deliver them who through fear of death were all their lifetime subject to bondage. 16 For verily he took not on him the nature of angels; but he took on him the seed of Abraham. Hebrews 2: 14 - 16

When I remember that healing is always available to me I begin to take my healing and deliverance from that attack in my body by faith. And sure enough healing always comes.

A Word in Season
GOD'S PLAN FOR YOU IS GOOD
"For I know the plans I have for you," declares the Lord, "plans to prosper you and not to harm you, plans to give you hope and a future"

2

You will not be put to shame

Jesus is the only reason that we have the hope of salvation. Salvation does not only mean to be born again, it means so much more than that.

When you became born again your Salvation came as a total package. God knew the things that you will have to face in life, He knew those things that will confront you and me as a person and he made provision for you in Redemption, if you can only believe.

This is what our Salvation Package brings to us:

Original Greek Translation of the word – <u>saved</u> – found in Romans 10: 11 - the verse of scripture that shows us how we receive salvation means:

- To save, keep safe and sound, to rescue from danger or destruction
- To save one (from injury or peril)

- To save a suffering one (from perishing), i.e. <u>one suffering from disease, to make well, heal, restore to health</u>
- To preserve one who is in danger of destruction, to save or rescue
- Save - make whole - Heal - be whole.

Take this truth and meditate on it until it becomes your reality, that you have been saved. Your salvation package came with healing, wholeness and soundness. So, we can make that withdrawal with our faith. We can take healing and deliverance by faith when attacked in any area of life or in our flesh, but ultimately, healing and health has been purchased for us so we can live in health as God's greatest desire for us which He says, "I wish above all things that you prosper and be in health even as your soul prospers" 3John 1: 2

You will not be put to shame

You have a guarantee from the same verse of Scripture in Romans 10: 9 11, the word of God says that you will not be put to shame. God and His Word are one, the word of God is God. You must take the word of God as God talking personally to you because that is exactly what it is.

I remember a period in my life that the enemy threatened me with symptoms and I clung to the word but I still did not come to that place of complete persuasion because faith is rest, when faith is present, we rest. But fear was still trying to take a hold on me and I would reach out to God by just physically looking up to heaven and I wanted something tangible that I could touch just to give me an assurance. One day as I longed for God and crying, He spoke from within me and said, "why are you looking up to heaven for me" He said, "look to the Word, the Word in your hand is God" that brought me great comfort and from that day, I began to see God in His Word as though He was right there because really, He is present with us by His word and by His spirit.

You see we look to God everywhere but in the Word. Don't get me wrong I am not saying that we do not go to the Word of God, we do but we are still looking for a physical manifestation of God to strengthen our faith. There is nothing wrong with that either.

What I am saying is that we can confidently look to the Word of God in our area of need and make that our confidence because that pleases God more. Jesus is the word of God made flesh. Don't forget that. The word of God is a "more sure word of prophecy" More sure and superior than any other evidence of God in our lives or this present world.

Anything else can be copied, the enemy can speak like an audible voice of God or speak through men like God or even appear like an angel, but he cannot corrupt the word of God. It is incorruptible. If you have ever desired to see and touch Jesus in that time of need, then know today that He is not far from you. He is in you by the Person of His Spirit and by His word in you and in your hand. Now that is great comfort.

Remember the Roman Centurion that came to Jesus making petition for one of his servants, Jesus immediately responds with compassion and said, "I will come with you" even though He had not yet physically paid the price for sin to give Him grounds to be a healer to the gentile. You remember that He is the Lamb of God slain from the foundation of the world.

The centurion and the gentiles were covered from the foundation of the Lord for Jesus to be their healer and deliverer. Showing us the mind of God for us. But the Centurion answered Jesus and said something very profound, and coming from a gentile, it greatly impacted Jesus and has left us believers a legacy of faith that should be based and founded only in the word of God and nothing else.

He gave an example to show Jesus that he perfectly understood what he was going to say and then he said to Jesus "Speak the word only" In response Jesus marveled and said, "I have not seen such great faith, no not in Israel" Matthew 8: 5 - 13 so faith in the word of God alone, Jesus says is qualified as "great faith" Think about that for a moment.

When we put our faith in the word of God, it is classified as "great faith" Faith in the Word of God is the highest level of faith and it is exactly the same as having faith in God. Jesus told the disciples that the Master key to the faith that moves mountain is faith in God, the same as faith in the word of God.

Now as you gave your life to Christ, at Salvation you have a guarantee that you will never be put to shame. This is what the scripture says;

> That if thou shalt confess with thy mouth the Lord Jesus, and shalt believe in your heart that God hath raised him from the dead, thou shalt be saved. 10 For with the heart man believeth unto righteousness; and with the mouth confession is made unto salvation. 11 For the scripture said,

whosoever believeth on him shall not be ashamed.
Romans 10: 9 -11

The Scripture above tells us and shows us the process of receiving salvation. That is how we got saved, by confessing the Lordship of Jesus Christ and believing in our heart that the Father has raised Him from the dead, and we are saved.

Then verse 11 says that "whosoever believes on Jesus will not be put to shame" when I saw this truth, I held unto it when the devil threatens me in any way, especially with symptoms in my body that refuses to go away. I stand on this word and keep declaring that I will not be put to shame because sickness and disease is shame and reproach to the believer.

I pray for you: In the same way I pray for you today that you will come out of that situation no matter how desperate it may be because the word of God is a sworn oath which cannot fail. You will not be put to shame; God is committed to bring His word to pass in your life. Again, I say that you will not be put to shame.

Apart from the total redemption of your person, your healing and deliverance came as a total package in salvation.

I would like to let you know up front that, that situation no matter how desperate it is, will not overcome you. Why can I speak so confidently? You may say at this point that, I have no idea how far gone this situation is, you may say, that if only I can see you now then I will understand how difficult things stand now, that report has no consequence, it will not leave a mark on you! Isaiah 43: 2 says so.

This is what this little epistle to you is all about. This book is written specially to you by the inspiration of the Holy Spirit so you will notice that it speaks directly to your heart. It is for you, the Lord put it in my heart to write this for you so that He can speak to your heart directly. So, open your heart and forget about that situation for a moment and put your gaze on Jesus. Look to Jesus, He is the author and perfecter of your faith.

The more you look to and give all your attention to your condition or situation, it takes the place of God, and it becomes your god. It will dictate to you how you live life, it will take the first place above everything else and God will become secondary as the condition allows. It should not be so.

I am not saying that all of this will come easy, but faith is an act of purpose, we exercise our faith on purpose. We do it anyway. When we give God His place by believing in His word, everything else will become subject to Him and begin to fade away. Hallelujah!

It means that Jesus will take your faith from where it is right now, that faith that has not produced for you that desired result, as you focus on Jesus, He merges your faith with His faith and the result must come, healing must come, breakthrough will come.

Close your eyes right now and see Jesus in any position you want to see Him. Maybe by your bedside, or sitting on the sofa with you or the kitchen table, in the garden, where ever, just see Him siting with you. I like to see Him wrap His arm around me enveloping me in His love as my Comforter and healer, my rescuer and deliverer and my Peace. He is my Shalom. Then open your eyes and open your heart and let the Word of God speak to that situation and bring to you the change you desire. I want you to dare to believe God now!

Release your faith now no matter how small and you will see the surge of power flow through to change that situation. You may not see immediate change but I can tell you that at the release of faith, just believe and don't doubt and the root of that situation, sickness or disease is already compromised at the instance of your flicker of faith. Now sit back and Jesus will speak into your heart. The Scripture tells us that:

> When the even was come, they brought unto him many that were possessed with devils: and he cast out the spirits with his word, and healed all that were sick:
>
> 17 That it might be fulfilled which was spoken by Esaias the prophet, saying, Himself took our infirmities, and bare our sicknesses. Matthew 8: 16 - 17

I want you to believe this because it is the truth. God does everything by His word only, and the faith that you need to stop that condition in its tracks so that it does not overcome you -- and to change that situation, or bring you that healing or deliverance and breakthrough is only found in the word of God.

Jesus healed and delivered by a word. The scripture tells us that as Jesus taught the power of God was present to Heal

The word of God comes equipped with the faith and power for your healing to happen for you now or for your desired breakthrough and turn around.

A testimony: I heard this testimony just today in Church; I believe that it is not a coincidence. This is for you.

A young man was diagnosed with cancer in his bladder, on receiving that report, He immediately set out and got a collection of faith messages and began to listen repeatedly. After a while, according to his testimony, he said, he spoke to his bladder and said, now you hear the word of the Lord I am playing this message for you to hear – you know that any form of sickness or disease is an offspring of the spirit of infirmity, so you are dealing with an intelligent being, be it disease, sickness or debt or a court case, or stagnation, lack or want, there are spirit beings working those things.

So, he went on to play the messages to his bladder and sure enough the spirit behind that condition must succumb to the preaching of the word of God, the condition was reversed. He was free from the infirmity of cancer in his bladder.

Now you may say, that was not very serious, but let me let you know, or remind you that the same faith that re-moves a head ache or a rash in the mildest form, is the same that will cure the worst state of cancer, heart disease or remove debts and bring financial breakthrough or what-ever it maybe.

Your condition no matter at what stage it may stand right now requires your little faith. Jesus said only believe to Jairus in the face of death, He said all I want from you now is stay in the place of faith and leave this to me. Don't give me fear now; give me faith to work with. Remember all that is required is your little faith to shift that mountain of debt, sickness and disease.

A Word in Season
BLESSED BE GOD

Blessed be God, even the Father of our Lord Jesus Christ, the Father of mercies, and the God of all comfort; 4 Who comforted us in all our tribulation, that we may be able to comfort them which are in any trouble, by the comfort wherewith we ourselves are comforted of God. 1Corinthian 1: 3 – 4

3

Your little faith can move that mountain

You may think that your condition is past the place of recovery, but let me show you that faith can reverse any situation.

The Disciples of Jesus were amazed that the fig tree that Jesus cursed the day before had dried up from the roots and withered away.

In response, Jesus gave us the number one key to dealing with the impossible. The number one Key to remove anything that looks immovable is;

The master key is "have faith in God"

The faith that makes the impossible to happen and reverse any situation, is the faith that is in partnership with God. Remember we has said that the Word of God is God exactly. When you take the word of God in any situation and stand on it in prayer that means you have invited God into that situation and you have come into agreement and partnership with the Word of God in your area of need. God now comes into active partnership with you to bring that word to pass for you. Mind you if someone comes to me and demands that I pay their child's tuition or pay of their mortgage or take on any kind of obligation that I did not promise them. I will not be obligated to meet that demand because I did not promise it.

But if I am a person of integrity and I have the means to be a blessing to someone and I made a promise to give a college scholarship to a family, then I become liable to fulfill that commitment because of my good name and standing in society.

God will only do for us what He has promised in His word. The good news is that the scripture says that "all the promises of God in Christ Jesus are yes and in Him amen" Jesus has paid the price for every promise that God has made to us in His word. The promise that "with His stripes you were healed" the price has been paid for that.

"He became poor that we through His poverty might become rich" the price has already been paid for you to live a rich full life. "I am come that you may have life and live it more abundantly" this price has been fully borne by Jesus Christ for you and me to live free from the oppression of the devil in sickness and disease, lack and want, shame and reproach, we are free to live the good life.

Do not fear, God will not disappoint you, He will not fail you. A dear servant of God would always say" God is too faithful to fail" and the Scripture says that;

If we believe not, yet he abides faithful: he cannot
deny himself. 2 Timothy 2:13

Believe in God

Jesus said again - with man it is impossible, but with
God all things are possible"

Jesus said to Martha "I have told you that – If you believe, you will see the Glory of God" that is if you believe,
you will see the power of God in manifestation.

When the man whose son had, epilepsy had come to the
end of himself and the disciples of Jesus at the time could
not help him, he went to Jesus and fell at his feet and said,
"Master if you can do anything, have mercy on me"

The Master rebuked him for his lack of faith, why did
Jesus do that? And then gave us another key to changing
any situation that confronts us. He said, "if you can believe, all things are possible to him that believes" He said
this simply because he expects us to believe God because
of all that we have seen and heard God do.

We have enough personal experience in our lives for us
to look back on and say, the God that delivered me from
so and so, is the same and He will do this one also. God
loves faith; it is a proof of our confidence and trust in Him.

God loves and responds to our faith at any time "without faith it is impossible to please God" if God is not
pleased with you, who will you turn to? We must believe
God no matter what and He will not fail us.

Jesus is saying to you now: if you can believe, all things
including that condition, anything, Jesus said all things irre-
spective of what it maybe, your own peculiar situation,
condition and circumstance is included in the "all things"
He said all things are possible to you if you can just believe.

Your ability to simply believe God and take him at His word, that is faith. And you know that you cannot get God to do anything for you, you cannot get Him to change your situation by feeling sorry for yourself and hoping that something will happen.

Faith is not passive; faith is an active participation with God as we engage His Word in any area and circumstance of our lives.

Without faith, we cannot please God. We must give God faith to work with. Faith applied correctly, as Jesus shows us in Mark 11: 23 - 24, cannot fail.

Faith can raise the dead

Jesus told His disciple that the key to getting results in life is faith in God. He spoke to the fig tree and it dried up from the roots and He said it is the result of faith in God and then He went on to show us how the entire process of faith in God works which is found in Mark 11: 22 – 24

> And Jesus answering said unto them, Have faith in God.
>
> 23 For verily I say unto you, that whosoever shall say unto this mountain, be thou removed, and be thou cast into the sea; and shall not doubt in his heart, but shall believe that those things which he said shall come to pass; he shall have whatsoever he said.
>
> 24 Therefore I say unto you, what things so ever ye desire, when ye pray, believe that ye receive them, and ye shall have them.

25 And when ye stand praying, forgive, if ye have
ought against any: that your Father also which is in
heaven may forgive you your trespasses.

Jesus lived and walked on this earth by faith in God, you
may say O but He is the Son of God, No He said we
would do greater works than He did as He returns to the
father. Why is that? how is it that we are supposed to do
greater works than Jesus?

He gave us the answer; He said that when He goes, the
Father will send the Holy Spirit, the comforter and the
spirit of Truth, the power of God to dwell with us and
abide with us forever.

The Holy Spirit is the Father in Jesus that was doing all
the works that Jesus did. He is also the Father in us doing
all the works and confirming the Word of God in our lives
and through us.

God will heal you, deliver you and make you free to experience the blessing so that He can use you to reach out
to many also.

Jesus used His faith to heal the sick, raise the dead and
set the captives free. The widow of Nain did not even
know who Jesus was, she was blind with grief because her
only son had just died but Jesus moved with compassion
used His own faith to restore her son to Her.

In the case of Mary and Martha, their brother was not
only dead, he had since been buried and corruption had set
in and yet the faith of Jesus reversed that situation and restored their brother back to them.

Your situation cannot be this desperate and even if it is,
your flicker of faith no matter how small if you plant it in
the Word of God it has the capacity to turn anything
round, it becomes "great faith" Hallelujah!

The faith of Jesus is available to you

In the book of Luke chapter 7 and verse eleven, we have mentioned earlier that the widow of Nain was too deep in grief to see or even notice Jesus, and He moved with compassion and stopped the burial procession and raise the dead man and restored him to his mother.

The woman did not supply her faith, so the compassion of God kicked in and Jesus supplied His faith. That was Jesus using His faith to bring relief to a grieving mother. Now, He had not yet gone to the Cross to pay the price for our victory and liberty. Now things are different, the price has been fully paid for you to be delivered from that affliction today, so take it now by faith. Believe you receive and it will be done to you according to your faith!

Jesus said; "lest at any time they should see with their eyes, and hear with their ears, and should understand with their heart, and should be converted, and I should heal them" Matthew 13: 15

What this means is that the day that the truth comes to you in your area of need and you receive it believe and understand it in your heart and have a change of heart, then He says, that same day, that same moment He will heal, and your change must come.

Today is that day for you, what this epistle is all about is to bring you to the place of full and absolute persuasion that God wants you healed now, delivered and set free from that oppression of the devil.

Another revelation that has been my strength is this truth that were my faith is weak and I tend to want to begin to doubt, I can switch to the faith of Jesus by saying it.

This truth came to me a few years ago I woke up from a dream and in that dream, I saw that I had a symptom in my body and as I woke up I was so distressed and I looked to the Holy spirit and He made this statement to me, He said "it would have been so, but Jesus Christ the Son of the living God loved you and gave Himself for you"

So, at any time the enemy threatens me with anything, the Lord reminds me of this truth and that removes fear and that is it. Apostle Paul in this Scripture that the Holy Spirit used shows us that there is a "faith of Jesus" available to us to live by. He said;

> I am crucified with Christ: nevertheless, I live; yet not I, but Christ lives in me: and the life which I now live in the flesh **I live by the faith of the Son of God**, who loved me, and gave himself for me. Galatians 2: 20

There is a faith of Jesus for you to reach out to right now if you think your own faith is weak or you do not have faith at this point to continue to stand. Mind you the widow of Nain did not even see Jesus let alone exercise her faith, so Jesus supplied His faith to give her what she did not even believe for or ask for.

There are many times that the Lord would do great things for me that even if I had to ask, my own faith would not have been able to carry that thing that He gave me or did for me, in a situation like that God Himself supplies the faith to give you that thing.

Now I pray for you: Father I ask that you supply your faith as confirmation of this truth not so that we live without faith but as an act of compassion to bring this child of

Abraham out of this difficult situation right now. Lord heal the sick, deliver the afflicted, intervene on our behalf and bring our desired breakthrough and turn around testimony. Lord in the end we will give all the Glory to you. In the miracle name of our Lord Jesus Christ amen!

Stay in the place of faith

You must do everything to stay in the place of faith. I love what Dr Bill Winston says. When he is standing in faith for anything, whether it be a need, a project or even a condition, he keeps everything that will bring doubt or distract him from his place of faith, he keeps such out of his life on purpose.

He said that one day, his wife came home and wanted to share something that had upset her and he said to her "not now sweet heart, I am working on something" Likewise the wife also does the same. You see they had the understanding that when they have any situation that they are standing in faith for, everything that can remotely oppose that stand of faith must be eliminated on purpose. You must learn to do that.

One of the ways is that you surround yourself with faith building messages, you do that purposely. If you know people who do not believe like you do and will speak or act in a way that will violate your faith, then you stay away from them for as long as you need to. Put yourself in an environment of faith in God on purpose. Put yourself in an environment of the word of faith so that your faith can be built up.

Jesus said to Jairus

Jesus said to Jairus in the face of his only daughter's death "fear not, only believe' meaning, don't give me fear now, stay in the place of faith and everything will be alright, just stay in the place of faith, it does not take anything to just believe. Believe God anyway. Just say like apostle Paul said, "I believe God" Dr Kenneth E Hagin said when he is threatened and pushed to the wall, this becomes his final place of faith and confession "I believe God'

Remember what the angel said to Daniel. He said, "Then said he unto me, fear not, Daniel: for from the first day that thou didst set thine heart to understand, and to chasten thyself before thy God, thy words were heard, and I am come for thy words: Daniel 10: 12. He said, "your words were heard and I have come for your words" think on this. He said in heaven your words, that is what you say is heard and heaven is going to respond based on what you say.

Why is this so important? That is because the angels of God who are the ones that do His bidding according to Psalm 103: 20 "they hearken unto the voice of His word" they excel in strength hearkening unto the voice of His word. So, you must be careful to store up the word of God in your heart so that this will become the only thing that comes out as you open your mouth when challenged in anyway. Store up the word in your heart on purpose. Gloria Copeland says, "no deposit, no return" think about that.

The scripture also says that in that dark place, you do well to pay close attention to the word of God because it is the light that will lead you out of that place. 2Peter 1: 19 also remember in that dark valley according to Psalm 23 it says that "I will not fear, for the Lord is with me, His rod and staff they comfort me' that is His word and His spirit is our comfort in every dark place in life. His word to comfort, and as light to show us the way out of trouble and His Spirit to comfort and guide us.

Do not mind the fact that, the angel said to Daniel that the Prince of Persia resisted him for twenty-one days that is why his answer was delayed. That is no more the case with us, for us "it is by faith that it might be by Grace so that the promise might be sure to all the seed" Romans 4: 16

For us "we are saved – healed – delivered – helped - blessed – prospered by Grace through faith as a gift of God so that no one may boast" Ephesians 2: 8. Our faith is that substance of the things we hope for and the evidence of the things that we have not yet seen. Hebrews 11: 1. For us our faith is now. For us we have the name that is above every other name and that name is our authority over the powers of darkness so if we live and operate by that name, the powers of darkness cannot resist or stop us as they did in the days of Daniel because at that time they did not have the name of Jesus to live by.

We have been told to do all in the name of Jesus Christ. So, we live by that name, which is "above every other name and at the mention of the name of Jesus, every knee should bow and every tongue confess that Jesus Christ is Lord to the Glory of God the Father" in our Lives.

As Jesus was with Jabirus, so He is with you and me by His word and spirit to Comfort and guide us out of any kind of situation in life. At this point, God supplies His faith to bring us through. Notice that Jesus took over at the point that Jarvis's faith could fail, Jesus supplied His faith. Even Jesus had to filter His own company and keep only those who would remain in the place of faith to accomplish the task ahead of them. So, work with Him today through the ministry of His word and His spirit and He will certainly without fail bring you out of that situation into your desired victory Hallelujah!

Use Your faith

The Master Key to your Turn Around Testimony

Your little faith can shift that large Mountain.

Now Jesus did not say that you can only change difficult situations when you can build up great faith. No, it is the application of your little faith - that is faith like the grain of mustard seed which is the smallest seed in the world – when you sow that faith as a seed the same way that a farmer would do just the way Jesus said, that small faith becomes great faith just because you have dared to use / sow it.

He said that Mustard seed which is like your faith when planted, grows to become a great shrub and the birds come and nest on it.

I recently heard Dr Yonggi Cho refer to this same statement by Jesus. He said that Jesus did not ask us to have great faith to change our situations or to root out that mountain. He went on to say that even if you have 1% faith out of 99% if you use that 1% it has the capacity to root out the mountain. That is phenomenal, think about that.

What does this tell us? Many times, we have the faith that can hand us our desire or give us our break through, but we just do not use it or maybe we do not know how to use our faith. We believe but we do not know how to engage with what we believe – which means putting our faith to work for us.

After you believe, you put your faith to work or use your faith by acting according to what you believe. It is when you dare to believe God and take that stand of faith to take your healing and deliverance that your faith becomes active and translates to great faith. Your little faith is energized on application with adequate power to shift any situation. Remember Jesus said, "all things are possible to the one that believes" if only you can dare to believe.

For example, the woman with the issue of blood heard about Jesus and all the mighty works that God was doing through Him, for Jesus had the testimony that "His fame grew abroad" she believed what she heard but did not stop there. She used all her strength to put action to her faith, that is, she planted her faith in what she believed by her action. As she did so, everything opened to her. Notice that she had to push through the crowd and no one stopped her, even the Jews who knew that coming out among the crowed with an issue of blood meant death by stoning, but her engagement of faith preserved her until she touched her point of contact.

Jesus said in that great chapter of faith

> For verily I say unto you, that whosoever shall say unto this mountain, be thou removed, and be thou cast into the sea; and shall not doubt in his heart, but shall believe that those things which he said shall come to pass; he shall have whatsoever he said.
>
> 24 Therefore I say unto you, what things so ever ye desire, when ye pray, believe that ye receive them, and ye shall have them.
>
> 25 And when ye stand praying, forgive, if ye have ought against any: that your Father also which is in heaven may forgive you your trespasses.
>
> 26 But if ye do not forgive, neither will your Father which is in heaven forgive your trespasses.

- If you believe, you should say to that mountain – be removed and be cast into the sea
- And shall not doubt in his heart - don't doubt!
- Believe that what you have said will come to pass – and it will.
- You will have whatever you say.

This is the pattern and prescribed order for us to see our desire come to pass for us.

We are a people who believe we receive

Recently this phrase came out of my spirit and began to speak to me. It said, "we are a people who believe we receive" and as I thought on this, it opened to me. As believers, we do not operate in any level of doubt. Apostle Paul said, "believing all things which are written in the law and in the prophets" Acts 24: 14

Jesus taught us how to receive from God every time in the Scripture above. He also taught us how to get results all the time. He said when you say what you want "believe and do not doubt in your heart. I heard Brother Kenneth E Hagin say "you can reason or doubt in your head, but do not doubt in your heart" Your head will reason and try to figure out how, but you must keep your heart firmly in the place of faith.

When your head reasons and try to produce doubt, we consciously block out doubt by believing what the Word says anyway. keep the promise of God in your area of need in your eye, in your ear, settling down in your heart, coming out of our mouth and it will feed your spirit and keep him strong to constantly supply you with faith. Keep hearing and hearing the word in your area of need, for instance we are taking our healing here so we keep the word of healing in our ear our eye and in our heart coming out of our mouth.

That is how you keep doubt out and remain in the place of faith while we give God time to perfect our desire and healing for us. Remember He is working behind the scene to bring your healing, deliverance and breakthrough.

We may not know how but we believe God anyway, you may not see anything happening, but you believe God anyway because we know that He is "working in us both to will and to do in us what is pleasing to Him" which is healing resulting to divine health. I also heard Dr Creflo Dollar say many years ago "God has more than a million and one ways to give us anything we want or to do for us what we desire of Him" think about that and if you try to figure that out, then that means frustration and it will lead to unbelief. So, what do you do? Jesus said only believe. That is all you and I are required to do. Believe only!

Jesus said that it is at the same time that you pray, as you are done praying, believe you receive the things that you have requested of God and you will have them. You do not wait until you see what you asked for physically before you believe, no it is when you pray that you believe you receive and you have it.

Jesus said something profound to Thomas after he was told that Jesus had resurrected and has even appeared to the disciples. Thomas said; "if I do not see I will not believe" So when Jesus appeared again among them before he went back to heaven, he specifically called Thomas to put his hand in His side and see that it was really Him Jesus. It is at this point that Thomas fell on his face and cried out "my Lord and my God" but Jesus was not impressed by that. This is the conversation between Jesus and Thomas that day; John 20: 26 - 29

And after eight days again his disciples were within, and Thomas with them: then came Jesus, the doors being shut, and stood in the midst, and said,

Jesus: Peace be unto you.

Jesus to Thomas: Reach here your finger, and behold my hands; and reach here your hand, and thrust it into my side: <u>and be not faithless, but believing.</u>

Thomas: My Lord and my God.

Jesus: Thomas, because you have seen me, you have believed: <u>blessed are they that have not seen, and yet have believed.</u>

Now the whole point of this section is that, in the world you would always hear the phrase "seeing is believing" you must understand that the world is running contrary to the Kingdom of God. We do not flow in the direction of the current; we swim upstream that is why it will take a **firm commitment** to live the life of faith. A dear servant of God said, "you cannot use the faith of Thomas to receive the blessing of Abraham"

What Jesus is showing us is that in the Kingdom of God is that - we believe to see. It is your ability to believe the Word of God that activates it and produce the anointing within to work for you, that is the power of God that the Word carries within it to produce what you want. Without this process, the Word of God remains dormant; yes, the word remains in-active and un-productive. That is why many lack results and then become discouraged. You believe you receive when you pray and you will have them. We are to believe we receive just as we pray.

The Holy Spirit said this to me many years ago, I had made a request to God and then I had put in an application to a Government agency and I prayed to God for favour. At that time, I was actively studying how faith works and I was reading Kenneth E Hagin's Books on faith. My head began to suggest that my application may not be granted and provided many reasons why it should be so and many good reasons and some very silly to believe reasons and yet it could create doubt, and as that kept happening and I stood my ground on the Scripture I heard the Holy Spirit say to me "what you have received, you do not yet hope for" that struck me.

He was referring to the Scripture in Romans 8: 26 which says, "For we are saved by hope: but hope that is seen is not hope: for what a man sees, why does he yet hope for?"

He used this Scripture in reverse. He said if you believe you received when you prayed, why are YOU now hoping that what you have already taken delivery of when you prayed will be granted at a future date? If you received it after you prayed, then it is already yours, it is already in your hand, you already have it, it is now yours. That request is now in your possession, it is done for you as you have prayed and believed for, all you are now expecting is the manifestation. You see what I mean?

Now on another occasion I also prayed and made request before the Lord and when I began to wonder in my head, notice that what your head does and what your heart does is different. You reason with your head how can this be done, but with your heart you believe unto salvation – you believe unto healing – unto deliverance and breakthrough. So, on this occasion the Holy spirit asked me a question this time, He said to me "Ema, did you believe you receive when you prayed" I began to think to myself did I do that or did I just pray and hope that something would happen when I prayed like many do and then doubt sets in and steals our answer to prayer and we keep going without results to back up our faith. We must be conscious to believe we receive when we pray – that is that your answer is ready at the same time as you pray, you do not wait for your answer, you receive it. Jesus said that our request in prayer is granted as we pray. Praise the Lord!

You must forgive

The very first thing to note is that forgiveness is for your own benefit in the first place. You must make up your mind to forgive even if the other person is unrepentant about what they have done, forgive anyway. Some people may not even know they have wronged you so in this case they cannot even come to say sorry, so if you keep that grudge who will suffer the consequence of it? because the person that wronged you is going about their business while you are bound in the chains of un-forgiveness and become unprogressive and may become sick in your body. Think about it, is it worth the trouble that it results in?

We cannot over emphasis this point, many in the body of Christ are sick and are in a prolonged state of illness and many go from one type of affliction to the other. The effect of un-forgiveness does not only result to sickness as science has proven repeatedly, it is also the root cause of every form of stagnation, limitation and lack of progress. Many are barren because there is a root of bitterness sitting deep in their heart because of un-forgiveness – relationships or past relationships.

The God that we serve is a spirit and only works by faith, for without faith, it is impossible to please God. Now the act of forgiveness is also an act of faith, you must engage faith to forgive. Why is that so? This book will not be complete if we did not deal with this aspect of our faith walk. Why do we need faith to forgive? Faith is not passive, you will not feel like walking by faith 100% of the time, so you must do it on purpose. Faith is like swimming against the tide, you are swimming upstream, contrary to the natural way of life "you call things that be not as though they are" so you should do it even when you do not feel like it because, I tell you, you will not. That is why Brother Norvel Hayes wrote the book "Faith has no feelings"

That is why it is written for us that we do not walk by sight but by faith. You will not want to forgive in many occasions, if the hurt and wrong is so bad that you will determine in your heart not to forgive. You hear many say

"I will never forgive that person" or "I will never forget" or yet still some say something like "I may forgive, but I will not forget" some even say that to their spouse or parent or children, and even to friends. You notice that I said in your heart, not in your head. So then un-forgiveness sits within the heart of a man. This is also the seat of faith and both cannot co-exist, one must give room to the other.

Faith is fed by the word of God, so if you will feed your spirit with the word of God and act according to what it says, then it will produce the faith to root out that un-forgiveness. You will also come to understand that if you do not forgive no matter what was done to you, you are holding yourself back and not the one that wronged you. That is why you must forgive so that you can move forward and your faith can produce for you.

We are called to keep the commandment of love and the lack of forgiveness is the opposite of love and faith works by love. Without Love in place your faith will not produce for you. That is why after Jesus gave us that great insight into faith and how we can receive from the father, at the end He added that we must forgive in the same way that the Father has forgiven us. It will take faith to forgive because as we have seen, faith does not operate by what we see, feel or touch, faith operates only by what God has said and that is final.

You must forgive no matter what, ask the Holy Spirit to search your heart if there be any root of bitterness because of un-forgiveness and then when He shows you, ask Him to help you to forgive. Then release your faith and take your healing and stand your ground. Faith will never fail you.

Use your mouth for your desired breakthrough

So essentially this portion of our receiving what we desire must come from our mouth. I tell you I know that in the face of difficult situations, you know what to say but find it hard to say it when the reality or facts stare you in the face.

It should obey you: Jesus said again: And the Lord said, if ye had faith as a grain of mustard seed, ye might say unto this sycamine tree, be thou plucked up by the root, and be thou planted in the sea; and it should obey you. Luke 17:6 -

Jesus described faith as seed, and by this we understand that if you leave a jar full of seed on your table for many years, like my father in the faith would say, it will remain as a seed, but if you cultivate the soil and plant it, then it will grow into a tree and into a forest and yield you the desired fruit.

Your faith becomes productive and fruitful when you sow it. Jesus is saying that we release our faith as seed sown into the soil by saying what we want, and then He gives us a guarantee that the situation will obey us.

I know that there are some situations that I know what to say but the reality before me makes my declaration of faith taste like chewing cardboard but as I say it over again, the anointing comes upon the word and at that point I know that in-spite of the physical appearance of things, the truth is that things have turned around and I will see the manifestation.

So, take the word of God in your area of need and say it in prayer, declare it to yourself, say it to anyone that you talk with and soon you will provoke the anointing to rest upon that word and the result will follow.

Many do not understand the relationship between the Word and the Spirit; this is how God does anything, that is by His Word and by His Spirit. Genesis Chapter 1 and John Chapter 1: 1-5 and at the birth of our Lord Jesus in Luke chapter one, this is how He does anything else. You work on the Word until the anointing flows out and activate that Word for you. You will know when this happens, it completely eliminates doubt. Faith is rest, you will know and things will begin to turn for good,

Many do not stay with the word – that is the promises of God long enough for the anointing to begin to flow out and activate the Word to make it productive so they give up on the letters which is logos. But rather as you stay with the written Word which is Logos the power comes on the Word and opens it up and it becomes Rhema that is when manifestation comes.

We do not and must never give up on the word of God, never! Jesus asked a question "when the son of man comes, will He find faith" Luke 18. Yes, he will find faith when He returns in my life and in your life. He said if we draw back from our faith, He will not be pleased with us, Hebrews 10: 38

Your faith has great reward and results attached to it so don't give up on the word of God no matter what the case is, the word can reverse it.

Hear what this Scripture is saying to you, please read it and believe. This caught me at the point that I was going to sink down into doubt and self-pity

> Cast not away therefore your confidence, which
> hath great recompense of reward. 36 For ye have

need of patience, that, after ye have done the will of God, ye might receive the promise.

37 For yet a little while, and he that shall come will come, and will not tarry. 38 Now the just shall live by faith: but if any man draw back, my soul shall have no pleasure in him. 39 But we are not of them who draw back unto perdition; but of them that believe to the saving of the soul.

Not too long ago I heard this scripture speak to me out of my spirit and that was the end of doubt and self-pity and I pulled myself up and said, all I need to do now is to give God faith to work with, and I got into the word to build my faith so that it can continue to come out of my heart and through my mouth. Then I began to consciously take actions that back up my faith – what I believe God for so that God can confirm His word for me. Glory to God forever!

5

Believe anyway

We have been told to look to our father Abraham and our mother Sarah, we must follow their faith. This is how Abraham believed for what God had promised him in the face of stack reality and the fact that they were up against an impossible situation naturally.

(As it is written, I have made thee a father of many nations,) before him whom he believed, even God, who quickens the dead, and called those things which be not as though they were.

18 Who against hope believed in hope, that he might become the father of many nations, according to that which was spoken, so shall thy seed be.

19 And being not weak in faith, he considered not his own body now dead, when he was about an hundred years old, neither yet the deadness of Sara's womb:

20 He staggered not at the promise of God through unbelief; but was strong in faith, giving glory to God; 21 And being fully persuaded that, what he had promised, he was able also to perform. 22 And therefore it was imputed to him for righteousness. Romans 4: 17 - 22

Faith is – turning and walking the opposite direction of what you see, feel, and know, but choose to believe God instead that is faith. Abraham's faith was strictly based on what God had said. "He believed according to that which was spoken, "so shall your seed be" He refused to allow his faith to become weak by his natural circumstance so he hoped and hoped repeatedly. Meaning that the promise of God was constantly before him, that is why he could keep his hope alive. I like the way a servant of God put it, he said "Abraham hoped and hoped and then he re-hoped" Meaning that he hoped and hoped and came to the end of himself and started all over again to hope. Think about that.

You must keep the promises of God in that situation in your eye and it will keep your heart from doubt and it can easily come out of your mouth so that it can be established for you.

Remember that it is the word you believe and declare that will be performed for you, not the one you believe and hid in your heart. Put it in your eye, your ear and it will settle down in your heart and become a garrison against doubt in the face of stack reality; it will flow from your heart to your mouth as you declare it in faith, that fact or reality must bow to the truth of God's word.

This was Abraham's reality and fact but He refused to stagger and give up on God and His promise to give Him a seed by Sarah." And being not weak in faith, he considered not his own body now dead, when he was about an hundred years old, neither yet the deadness of Sara's womb"

Please don't give up on God, all He wants is your faith, stand your ground and your Salvation will produce your desired breakthrough, healing or deliverance. Glory to God!

He could there do no mighty works

Without faith, the power of God is limited or becomes inactive. Our faith in God and in His word, is what activates the power of God. Jesus went back to His home town and could not do any mighty works there because of their lack of faith. This was because they knew Him and it was hard for them to go past that to see Him for who He truly is – the Saviour – Messiah, the son of God manifesting the power of God so they could not believe.

Many times, our solutions in life come in the way that we least expected, it may come from someone we can easily look down on. That is why God only gives Grace to the humble and resist the proud. Unbelief apart from being a direct result of ignorance, a lack of knowledge and understanding, is often an act of pride.

The proud would want God to do things for them in a certain way and outside of that, they get offended. The cure for unbelief is to seek knowledge and then we must check our heart with the help of the Holy spirit to see if there be any root of pride and then receive help to root out that pride so that you can humble yourself under the mighty hand of God.

> And he could there do no mighty work, save that
> he laid his hands upon a few sick folk, and healed
> them. 6 And he marveled because of their unbe-
> lief. And he went around about the villages,
> teaching. Mark 6: 5

Jesus did not give up on His kinsfolk though, He was not offended at them, but rather He went about the towns and villages and taught them. Dr David Oyedepo says that "every man's mountain is his ignorance" think about that for a moment.

Jesus said that "you will know the truth and the truth will make you free. In other words, it is the truth you do not know that will keep you in bondage. Whatever the condition is, all that is required is the knowledge of the truth concerning that situation. What has God said about it? Have you bothered to find out what the truth says about it? Or are you ignorant still? Have you chosen to remain ignorant still?

Jesus said that only one thing is needed. In any situation that confronts us, only one thing is needed and that one thing is the word of God in that area of need. If it is heal-ing, then only one thing is needful and that one thing is the Word of God on healing. What provision has God made for you, what promises have you found? How are you building your faith in that area of your need?

Every affliction, sickness, disease, debt, lack, want any kind of oppression, marital difficulties, limitation. Name it, whatever the case is and what ever stage it maybe, it all proceeds from that power of darkness, it is not of God. God will not partner with the devil to afflict His children that He paid a high price to redeem from the power of darkness.

King David said, "before I was afflicted, I went astray" He did not say God afflicted him; he took responsibility and looked to God to deliver him as he turned from any wicked way.

The scripture says that "how God anointed Jesus Christ of Nazareth with the Holy Ghost and with Power who went about doing good and healing all that were oppressed of the devil for God was with Him" Acts 10: 38.

That statement shows God in active partnership with His Son Jesus by His spirit to heal and deliver those oppressed of the devil, then what sense would it make for Him to go back to the devil to borrow his tools to afflict his children when they do wrong and sometimes do nothing at all just to teach them a lesson as some allude to.

What Father would do that? It is His goodness that brings us to the place of repentance, not His judgment, it is also His good pleasure to give us the Kingdom. Think about that. If God works with the devil in that way, then His Kingdom will be divided against itself.

You see what I mean. God wants you to come to the place of the knowledge of the truth so that you can give Him faith to work with and He can partner with you through faith to bring you out of that situation and you can serve Him. That is His vision and goal for us.

He taught them

Jesus went about teaching. What does that say to us? When their unbelief cut off the power of God so that Jesus could not, notice that it did not say that he refused to do, but "he could not do any mighty works except heal minor aliments" He knew the solution was in the lack of knowledge. Pride and unbelief are all a product of ignorance.

If you or any person knew better, they will humble themselves. God resist the proud and gives Grace to the Humble, so why will I want to stay on the wrong side of God, I would rather have God partner with me always that way my victory is guaranteed and if all it requires is my humility then I throw away anything that represents pride as He shows me.

A dear servant of God said that "every problem in life is a lack of wisdom" Knowledge is the answer to any challenge in life, when you know what the problem is and find the answer then the problem is solved.

So, knowing this, Jesus went about the towns and villages and taught them. Why, so that He could change their unbelief to faith through knowledge. Faith comes by hearing and hearing by the word of God. Romans 10: 17.

Everyone that came to Jesus and received their healing and deliverance, came to Him because Jesus had the testimony that "his fame grew abroad" they heard about Him and the power of God working through Him and they believed what they heard and put action to their faith by going to meet with Jesus and they all had that basic ingredient to our change of story which is that **they heard, believed what they heard and then took action.**

Going to Jesus is the exact same thing and has the same effect and result as going to the Word - the Word is Jesus and Jesus is the Word of God made flesh.

As they went to Jesus and got their deliverance we can by the Holy Spirit go to the Word and sure enough our healing deliverance and breakthrough must come. Glory to God!

6

What you should dare to believe

He sent His Word and healed them and delivered
them from their destructions Ps 107: 20

That surely, Jesus – the Word; has borne our
griefs and carried our sorrows.... And He was
wounded for your transgression, bruised for your
iniquities, the punishment of your peace was upon
Him and with His Stripes, you were Healed. Isaiah
53: 4 – 5 Matthew 8: 14 – 17, 1 Peter 2: 24

Do you believe this?

Jesus asked the two Blind men that cried out to Him for
mercy; do you believe that I can do this?" And they answered straight way "yes Lord" and immediately, Jesus
gave them a blank Check. I like to show you this release of
power for turn around and breakthrough, promotion res-

cue, recovery, deliverance and healing and whatever inter-vention we desire of God, I will show it in a different translation than King James which most of us are familiar with. It says:

> When Jesus got home, the blind men went in with him. Jesus said to them, "Do you really believe I can do this?" They said, "Why, yes, Master!"
>
> Jesus touched their eyes and said, "Because of your faith, you will be healed." - CEV
>
> Then he touched their eyes and said, "Because of your faith, it will happen." - NLT
>
> He touched their eyes and said, "Become what you believe." - MSG Matthew 9:29

I particularly like the Message translation. Jesus touched their eyes and said, "become what you believe" It is so true in every sense of that statement that you really become what you believe. It is as you think, so you become. It will always be to you according to your faith – that is your abil-ity to believe God and take Him at His word and act on what you have believed.

You can look up this Scripture in as many translations as you want for more clarity, which is what I do. Dr David Oyedepo puts it this way, he says "you can have it the way that you want it" because you have believed. **We must dare to believe God** that He will do for you as you have believed Him for and that He will do for you what He has promised in His word. It is this process of our faith that activates the power of God. Many wait for God to just show up and do something but do not realize that it is your faith, I did that for many years, oh the shear frustration, until God sent me teachers who brought me out of that rut. As you take the word of God in your area of need and go to God in prayer believing, that act of faith in God and acting accordingly is what will bring about our desired need.

Do you believe that He can do this?

This is a question that Jesus is asking everyone that come to Him seeking mercies of God in any difficult situation. He is asking you the same question right now and your answer will determine the outcome of His response to you. You see faith allows us to call the shots with God. When Jesus asked the two blind men in Matthew 9: 27 – their immediate response was "yes Lord" and His immediate response was "have it the way you want it" Glory to God!

Just a day ago I came face to face with this truth. My son who is eleven years was set to travel to Portugal to play in the under eleven world cup. This plan has been in place for the last one year and was been ongoing. We were all excited when the time drew near. It cost us a lot of money in preparation and finally the time had come. A day before they were due to travel on a Sunday morning, I woke the children up as usual and I went back to get ready for the Church service. As I checked they did not seem to be ready and my son that was due to travel with his team the next day was lying on the couch. He had woken up with upset stomach vomiting and faint.

I knew that I needed to begin to stand my ground. I took the seed that I had prepared to sow for the trip in my hand and I left for Church, I offered it to the Lord and after the service I got home believing that as I came back I would find him running around as usual, but this time that was not the case, the situation persisted. Through the day he was not eating and I panicked. He was running very high temperature and my focus was to keep him stable and comfortable.

I had the trip in mind and got into agreement that God will intervene and he would make the trip which was scheduled for the next morning. Through the night we battled to keep his temperature stable. I was in between if I should take him to the emergency room when the temperature became very high. I gave him cold showers and medication and I kept declaring the counsel of God, pleading the mercy of God in case I had done anything that opened the door for the enemy to come in and attack us that way.

To cut a long story short, it was a battle all through that night, **but I put on God like a garment.** He was in me and was with me and I listened intently for His voice every step of the way. I determined that the enemy will not steal from us what God had given us by His grace alone. When I enquired of the Lord many times through the night and said – Lord it is what you want that will happen here, as good as that sounds, the response I got back all the time which is a great experience for me was "it is what you decide"

It does not depend on what God wants in any situation we find ourselves in, it is what we decide that God will now put His weight behind and make happen for us. So, I got into agreement with my children that Joshua will make the trip. I kept administering the Communion table and declaring the Covenant of Peace which you will see at the end of this book.

I engaged the ministry of the Blood of the Covenant because I knew that this is my advantage over any attack of the devil for "we overcome him by the Blood of the Lamb" I would shower him and use the anointing oil to anoint him all over. I also prayed over water and black currant that I use for the Blood as the Blood of the Covenant in that bowl that speaks in Zion and I would sprinkle him with that to neutralize any negative thing around.

I also made sure that even though I was in panic mode because the clock was ticking, I made sure that my heart was full of faith, I believed God and kept the word of God in my eye coming out of my heart to my mouth. I kept feeding my faith. I knew that it is with my faith that I overcome the world – that is any adversarial condition. Your faith will overcome for you in any situation you come up against.

Like the woman with the issue of blood, I pressed on as the morning came with my eye set on bringing him to their meeting point. I said in my heart that if I stabilize him and get to the meeting point, I have exercised my faith, and things would turn and if it does not then I will go back home. The Scripture says when the four friends- tore the roof of the house that Jesus was in and dropped their friend through in front of Jesus, it says "and Jesus seeing their faith" which means that we must show our faith as we move decisively towards what we want God to do for us.

If I allowed myself to sit back overwhelmed and crying to God and running all over the place, we would have lost that wonderful Grace that God himself gave us. So, I continued to take care of that child through the night until morning and he began to stabilize and recover and was excited to meet up with his team mates. I had also laid out his club gear to motivate him to fight with me so he fought

51

too. Keep something in front of you that will motivate you to fight.

In that condition, what do you want to see happen, keep it in front of you. Bring out pictures of how you want to see yourself healed and healthy and keep that in front of you. Even if it is not your own picture, find an image that portrays what you want and that will keep you fighting for what you have before the Lord and then keep doing something to move you towards that and at the end, your vision will speak, it will answer for you and hand you their desire.

Sure enough as we got to the meeting point, every symptom disappeared and Joshua ate and was excited to meet up with the team to make the trip. I had gotten ready early enough and began to prepare telling myself and telling Joshua that we must give God faith – I kept saying within me that I must give God something to work with, He had to see my faith.

In between that night I would lie down for an hour or two and believed God for sleep because I also knew that God works when we rest. When we rest in time of crisis, it is an indication of absolute trust in the God we serve who has said "stand still and see the Salvation of the Lord" the one who has also said [this is my favorite one] "because you have set your love upon me, I will deliver you, I will be with you in trouble and I will deliver you and honour you and show you my Salvation" Psalm 91: 14 – 16 So God is in active partnership with us in any situation we find ourselves in and His ultimate mission is to deliver and bring you and me out with honour and to show us His Salvation which is translated to mean;

This word salvation comes from the Hebrew word - Y@shuw`ah – that is Saviour

Definition: Salvation, deliverance, Welfare, Prosperity, Deliverance. Salvation (by God), Victory

Our Saviour Jesus is saying right now - <u>I will show you my Salvation</u> – Meaning - I will;

    Save you, you will be saved, you will be delivered

    You will be liberated, be saved, be delivered

    You will be saved (in battle), be victorious

    I will save from moral troubles

    I will give victory to you

    Greek Equivalent Words: salvation, help, deliverance, health, save, saving, welfare

When you are confronted with a situation like the one I experienced, be it a prolonged situation or an intense one that I faced that was time sensitive, your mind will put pressure on you, you will begin to feel the pressure of condemnation of times you have been outright dis-obedient to what God wanted you to do. You begin to see what you may have done wrong to open the door for this attack. For me sure enough I was a bit distracted as I realized that Joshua's passport that I had applied for may not come back to me on time for the trip, I thought I had left it too late.

God gave me a testimony there because with a severe backlog with applications for the summer holiday approaching, it was near to impossible to get through to the passport office by telephone, **but by faith** I rang and the second time someone answered and I told them the need to have the passport ready and immediately they prioritized the issuance of the passport, but I was called and told that we had made a mistake that is why they did not process on time so I had to run around and send all the documents back and I found great favour with the person that was assigned specially to us and within two days, the passport was issued and sent to us by post.

Now this goes to also show that we were under attack of the enemy as the Lord gave us this good thing. I always make it a point to check by the Holy Spirit in any situation to see how I contributed to bring any situation about, so that I do not repeat the same mistakes. I do not assign blame to the devil immediately when things go wrong because he can only take advantage of the access we give him, many blame the devil for their foolishness and oversight instead of quietly admitting their error and seeking God to show them were they might have done something wrong. This is a sign of meekness and humility and strength of character before God. And the Scripture says that God reveals His secrets to the one that is meek, this is the place of great advantage in life. Now this is what I identified as my error:

- I allowed myself to be distracted
- I ought to have found out about the dates of travel earlier and put that in front of the Lord on my prayer alter daily
- Take three days before the trip to go into a fast which is something I would have done naturally but as I said, I was distracted.

What I did do right:
- I sowed a seed for the trip
- As we came together to pray our prayer group prayed over the trip many times.

What to do differently

This is unique to my situation but it applies to every situation, quit putting everything on the devil or you will go nowhere in life, learn to take responsibility and the devil will be in awe of you and you will win all the time. When you identify your mistake, run to God for mercy, I have found that place in Him and that is where I live – the place of His mercy. See Hebrews 4: 16. We will visit this place in a later chapter.

My son Joshua did make the trip with his team mates; I did not get to go with him though, which is another thing completely as I look at it now. I did not use my faith or put my faith where it ought to be to work for me, so we did not go as a family because I did not reach out to God consistently enough for the provision to do so. As I think of it now, my faith was sort of "flaky" if there is a word like that; Novel Hayes uses that a lot to descried inconsistent faith. The scripture says that we cannot receive anything from the Lord if we have "flaky faith" that is undeceive if we are double minded.

We must be focused and specific in our faith and the exact result we desire will come. It is all based on trust. All I thought at the moment was our plan to relocate to another country which is a major move and that consumed my thoughts and informed my decision to go with the plan that Joshua should go to the tournament with the team. As I think of it now, the Scripture says that "our God will supply all our needs according to His riches in Glory by Christ Jesus" Philippians 4: 19 He did not say some or part of our needs but all. So, I could have believed God to not only supply the provision for us to make that trip as a family but also to take care of everything we need for the plan to relocate from our present location.

Think about that so that the next time you had to believe God and it seems that it is too much, that there are just too many things to believe for all at once, remember put everything on the table and take a stand of faith and make your plan decisively towards your goal – that is what you are believing God for and God will not disappoint your faith for faith never fails. He will work with you and for you to do for you according to your faith.

We waver in our faith because we do not trust that God will do for us what we desire or need, while all the time it is what we believe and dare to take a stand for that God will do. It does not depend on God because it is always to you, according to your faith! We call the shots by faith and not God! So, I missed out on what was a wonderful experience to have our family together and for Joshua to have his family with him for support as other members of the team [three out of ten players went without their parents] simply because I did not, not could not but I simply did not focus my faith enough to receive, I allowed myself to vacillate between two opinions and that robbed me of my blessing to go and watch my son play on a world platform like that.

When I rang the coach when they had arrived Portugal from our location of Ireland, I spoke with Joshua and He was fine and so excited. He went on a trip that was at least a total of four hours and he was perfectly ok. These were the words of his coach when I first spoke to him as they arrived "Josh is fine. He seems very happy" that was good enough for me, Joshua is a striker and He scored wonderful goals for the team and I return all the Glory to God!

A Word in Season
THE LORD OUR DELIVERER

He shall deliver thee in six troubles: yea, in seven there shall no evil touch thee.

Job 5: 19

Because thou hast made the LORD, which is my refuge, even the most High, thy habitation; 10 There shall no evil befall thee, neither shall any plague come nigh thy dwelling. Psalm 91:9 – 10

7

Mercy will turn things around for you

Lord Stretch forth your hand to Heal now

Can we as believers pray and ask God to heal us even if the Scripture says that "with His Stripes, we were healed"? Putting our healing in the past tense as a finished work of God in Christ. The answer to this is yes. This is found in Acts 4:30 after Jesus died, resurrected and the Holy Spirit was sent, the disciples prayed and asked the Father to stretch forth his hand to heal and that signs and wonders be done in the name of His Holy Child Jesus. The response of the Father was instant with great evidence.

I was in a prayer meeting a while ago I had a discomfort in my body that just stayed there for so long and in that meeting, the Minister said, "ask the Lord to touch you and heal you right now" I always listen to prayer lines to see if it lines up with Scripture. Also, if what we are praying for has already been completed in the finished work and given to us to receive by faith instead of continuing to ask and make a request before God for what He has already given us.

As I enquired in my heart, immediately I heard in my spirit "the prayer that the disciples prayed in Acts 4: 30" and I went to check it out. They prayed and asked the Father to stretch forth His hands to heal as they went about preaching with boldness and that signs and wonders be done though His Holy child Jesus. Acts 4: 30 They were going out to minister to preach Christ and so they asked the Father to heal as Jesus said, "and these signs will follow them that believes, in my name they will lay hands on the sick and they will recover" Mark 16: 15 – 20

What that said to me is that we can still pray and ask the Father to stretch forth His hand to heal us, we can also as believers receive our healing that has already been given though Christ Jesus and enforce it in our situation so that like it is written in Matthew 8: 17 we can also say that we receive our healing and deliverance from any kind of affliction, so that it may be fulfilled for us that which was spoken by Isaiah the Prophet: himself took our infirmities and bore our sicknesses.

I invite you to say that now – say this as simple as it may sound, it is very powerful. Say and keep saying - I take my healing and deliverance now – [from so and so] that it may be fulfilled in my life that which was spoken by Isaiah the Prophet – Himself took my infirmities and bore my sicknesses. That word covers anything that you may be going through right now. Jesus Christ has paid a high price for all our mistakes and short comings.

Faith Rest

Another very important thing to note is that when we come under attack in any way, be it physical, financial or emotional or in our relationships, the first thing that will happen is that if we are not trained, panic will set in, there is nothing really wrong with that but we have to be very quick to get into the place of faith and stay there, if you continue to allow panic, fear will result and that will drain your faith and you need faith for God to move on your behalf.

We have said that "faith is an active partnership with God to accomplish the impossible" when we exercise our faith in God and in His word, we are essentially giving God an open invitation to come into that situation to partner with us, save us and bring deliverance from that situation. **The proof of faith is rest**. When you are not peaceful in that situation, you are not in the place of faith, so what do you do?

You must go on purpose to the faith bank and collect faith so that you can give God something to work with, so you can give God something to confirm for you. He said, "you shall decree a thing and it shall be established unto you" what do you want God to establish for you? If you panic you cannot think straight and you will not be able to hear the Holy Spirit, if you can't hear Him, how can he lead you out of that situation? How will He show you the way of escape from that situation?

As you get in a position of faith, rest comes. As you rest also on purpose in spite of all, faith will come also. How do you get faith? By going to where faith is stored, to where faith is produced and you will get faith to give God access into your situation. The Scripture says that "faith comes by hearing and hearing by the word of God" faith comes as we hear and continue to hear the word of faith in our area of need. If you need healing keep hearing the word of faith for healing, get anointed messages on healing and keep it in your eye, keep the Word of faith on healing in your eye and in your mouth. I keep it very simple for myself and for my family, we stay in Isaiah 53: 4-5 and then we can reference Matthew 8: 17, Psalm 107: 20, Proverbs 4: 22, and 1 Peter 2: 24.

For finance, we sow according to 2 Corinthians 9: 8 – 14 and we reference; Philippians 4: 19, Isaiah 30: 23 - 24, Zachariah 8: 12 Luke 6: and we receive our harvest back on the sport according to Amos 9: 13 -15 and We sow into Jesus our great High Priest who is the Lord of the Harvest who will watch over our harvest and will not allow the fowl of the air to plunder our harvest.

For answer to prayer you pray according to the will of God which is the Word of God, 2 John 5: 14 -15 This is first thing to do, you are to go into the Word which shows you what the will of God is in that situation, and then you take it to God in prayer. We have a guarantee right there that "if we pray according to His Will He hears us and if He hears us, then we have our petition granted" when you find what God has said in His word, we commit Him to confirm it and perform it for us. We said earlier that even you and I will only be obligated to perform or do for any-one what we have personally promised and are capable and trust worthy enough to fulfill what we promised.

That is why it is said that, Abraham "believed according to that which was spoken, so shall your seed be" that was the grounds of His faith, what God had promised not some random thing from nowhere. What promise are you standing on? Stay there and it will not fail you! It is said that Sarah "judged God faithful who had promised" Sarah took the promise and processed it against the one that had said it. Is He capable to perform what He has promised? Is he reliable? Can He be trusted? Can we invest our energy and emotions to believe Him? Does He have the resources to back up His word? And at the end the conclusion is that "she judged Him faithful" so our faith can only be based on what God has said, when you come into this place of faith, rest comes naturally and that Word takes over and begins to self-fulfill and reverse that situation for you.

Give Jesus faith to work with

We are instructed by scripture to labour to enter this place of rest which is the place of faith. Faith rests. There is no fear or apprehension in faith, if there is then there is no faith or your faith has been compromised so go after faith and remain there for "the just shall live by his faith" Habakkuk 2: 4, Romans 1: 17, Galatians 3: 11, Hebrews 10: 38, Jesus said to Jairus in the face of death "fear not, only believe" what I got from this is that Jesus said to him, don't give me fear now, give me faith, continue to believe, that is stand your ground for me, and from that point we see Jesus take over the situation and replace Jairus's faith with His own faith to overcome the spirit of death.

Remember when Jairus first went to Jesus He had declared his faith in the power of God working in Jesus. It is said that "He besought him greatly, saying, my little daughter lies at the point of death: I pray thee, come and lay thy hands on her, that she may be healed; and she shall live". Mark 5:23 – Jesus wanted him to remain in this place of faith that he had first exercised so that Jesus could work on

His behalf. Many people had gathered at this point in Jairus' home and in this kind of scenario, your faith can and will come under severe pressure, you go and see what Jesus did and do the same. 1) He sustained faith by removing and restraining fear. 2) He eliminated on purpose every source of doubt and unbelief. 3) He filtered His own company and only kept the ones that were in agreement with Him to perform this miracle. 4) He removed by standers and only kept those immediate family that had a vested interest in the outcome of His presence i.e. the parents and grandparents. Keep close family members and a close circle in the church to stand with you in faith for your desired victory.

When a situation that requires God's, intervention is thrown to the public scrutiny, it drains out the very ingredient required to deliver the solution, which is faith and many wonder why God did not move on their behalf. God is a faith God He requires our faith, that is for you to "believe only" so that He can move for you.

Do not cast your peal to the swain, don't go about telling everyone your situation, filter your company, keep company with those that have like faith and will stand with you in faith and in prayer and, those that have a vested interest in your total recovery and restoration like close and immediate family We must learn this vital lesson of recovery and victory over challenges from Jesus our Lord and Saviour. Pleased read all the book of Mark chapter 5 and it will bless you.

A word in Season
MERCY WILL CHANGE EVERYTHING

Behold, the eye of the LORD is upon them that fear him, upon them that hope in his mercy; Psalms 33:18
The LORD takes pleasure in them that fear him, in those that hope in his mercy. Psalms 147:11

Excerpt

"If you panic, then you cannot think straight and you will not be able to hear the Holy Spirit, and if you can't hear Him, how can he lead you out of that situation? How will He show you the way of escape from that situation?" Have faith in God for - Faith Rests.

8

Absolutely no Fear

Y ou must not fear! I was in a meeting recently and we were talking about the absolute importance of faith for the believer especially in these last days. Jesus said that "the heart of men will fail for fear" and that "many will fall away from the faith" He further questioned and said, "when the son of man comes will He find faith"?

That is something that you must be conscious of. And that is a serious question that we ought to search our heart to answer. If you find yourself wanting, it is time to remedy that by building your faith in God on purpose. We must see fear from God's perspective that way we will understand why He says fear not so many times in the Scriptures. Fear is not of God in any way. Fear first came with the devil in the garden of Eden. When Adam fell to sin and God came calling for him, when He heard the voice of God, he hid himself.

You see the first thing that fear does, it brings you under condemnation and makes you to hide from God so that God cannot help you. Now Adam said this to God when God called for Him after he fell into sin, he said "I heard thy voice in the garden, **and I was afraid**, because I was naked; and I hid myself" Genesis 3: 10

That is how fear came into the world through sin. But God has ransomed us, He has redeemed and justified us through His son Jesus Christ and the Scripture says that;

> There is therefore now no condemnation to them which are in Christ Jesus, who walk not after the flesh, but after the Spirit. 2 For the law of the Spirit of life in Christ Jesus hath made me free from the law of sin and death. Romans 8: 1 - 2

Now the point I want you to know and keep in mind is that God does not want you to fear, when He says fear not, it literally means "I have your back so trust me on this" Now God was angry with Israel for not believing Him when He told them to go in and take their promise land which is like you and I now. This is what the Scriptures says about that, "Whereby are given unto us exceeding great and precious promises: that by these ye might be partakers of the divine nature, having escaped the corruption that is in the world through lust" Peter 1: 1- 4

The Scripture says that you and I have "exceeding great and precious promises" and yet many are going about in pathetic conditions because they have no clue what Salvation has brought them. They have not been taught and are not able to release their faith to receive from God so they continue to go without and afraid of the devil and the powers of darkness.

God calls the one that fears 'evil" He says you have an evil heart when you do not believe what God says to you in His Word. When you do not trust, that God will rescue you, when you do not trust and put your faith in God and take steps to do what He wants you to do according to your faith, then God says You are like the unbeliever. You are evil. If you do not believe God as a Christian to help you and believe Him to do for you what He has promised, then you have gone from being a believer to becoming an unbeliever, you have fallen from Grace. This is how serious this thing is.

When you fear, it means you do not trust God to do His part for you. When you fear, you have taken sides with the devil and you are opposing God because He is not to be trusted, think about that because if we trust Him then we will not be afraid. I like the way King David deals with fear and I have adopted this and made it my place of refuge from fear. He says:

> What time I am afraid, I will trust in thee. 4 In God I will praise his word, in God I have put my trust; I will not fear what flesh can do unto me.

This is another Scripture that holds me up when fear wants to take hold of my heart, I will say this continually until that fear is broken:

> Behold, God is my salvation; **I will trust, and not be afraid**: for the LORD JEHOVAH is my

> strength and my song; he also is become my salvation. Isaiah 12: 2

The enemy will accuse God before you and bring you to the place of doubt. That is what He did to Eve, He said "did God say" that immediately begins to make you think again, you will begin to see how that so and so believed and yet nothing happened, or did they? You will begin to rationalize and see why the opposite can happen instead of what you believe for. You see why God does not want you to entertain fear at all. The enemy wants you to doubt God, He wants you to fall out of favour with God by your doubt which God hates so that with God working against you, they enemy can then have room to keep you in bondage and accomplish his mission which is to kill steal and to destroy.

The Scripture says that fear has torment. Fear will torment you if you allow it, it is the devils tool so it carries torment, it torments its victim. Think about that so you will not submit yourself to fear but rather you should trust God knowing that He will not fail you. When your faith is weak and fear wants to come, switch from faith to trust and rest. Trust is absolute dependent on God's faithfulness, and that is when the faith of God takes over for you. You hand it all over to Him and He will supply the faith to bring you out of that situation.

Fear gives the enemy something to work with, fear is a tool of the enemy, fear is the access that the enemy requires to establish his plan which is to kill, steal and to destroy. But on the other hand, as we have seen earlier, faith activates the power of God and brings God on the scene to partner with you and bring you out of that undesirable situation.

Now we must understand the origin of fear and the consequence of fear. I have absolutely no place for fear, I may panic but I take a stand of faith and consciously resist fear. Fear means I do not trust God, fear means that God cannot be trusted, Fear means that God is uncertain, we do not know if our stand of faith will hold out or fail us. What is faith anyway? Because if your faith is genuine, that is based on what God has said, then we have a sworn oath that it will not fail.

The word of God is first a promise and then it was established by a Covenant in the Blood of our Lord Jesus Christ and then God confirmed it by an oath. How secure do you want this thing to be? 2 Peter 1: 19 says the word of God is a "more sure word of Prophecy" therefore it is failure proof, it is an incorruptible seed. If you are trusting on the word of a man, it may fail you. But God's word abides forever, it cannot fail, no matter how feeble your faith in God is in the face of adversity, believe Him anyway and I guarantee that the Word cannot fail. The Word is God so how can He fail you.

Some people assume their faith and then they say, "I believed and it did not work" You do not try faith, faith is based on what God has said and you do not try the word of God, the Word of God has already been tried seven times by fire. It is pure and incorruptible, it is the word that will try you to see if you will stand your ground and believe God in spite of all.

How can it not work? Faith always works because it is always based only on what God has said, not on some presumption, not on any other person's experience, but only on the Word of God, what God has said in His word by revelation to you as a person, seeing that you must work out your own Salvation. Many have weak faith because they think or have heard of some believer that something negative happened to, but they quickly forget that it is always unto you according to **your own ability to believe** God and stand your ground upon His Word not according to what someone else experienced. You must work out your own personal Salvation with fear and trembling.

Fear will put you out of God eternal plan

What a lot of believers do not realize is that, Jesus is not only telling us "fear not" just to calm us and bring comfort in the time of trouble, but fear has and eternal consequence. When I saw that, I purposed in my heart that I will not allow fear into my heart. I will rather trust God and put my faith in Him trusting that:

- He will not allow me to be tempted with more than I can bear
- He has made a way of escape for me
- He has said that no evil will befall me
- He will be with me in trouble and deliver me and set me on high [lift me above that situation and the consequence of it] I will call on Him and He will answer me and deliver me, satisfy me with long life and cause me to see His salvation.
- He has borne my grief and carried my sorrows, therefore I will not grief and I will not sorrow, and no one will sorrow over me.
- I have been ransomed from the power of the grave
- I have a Covenant of peace established in the Blood of the everlasting Covenant
- My salvation and redemption guarantees that I will not be put to shame -

Now I can go on and on. This applies to you and every other believer that cares to believe for themselves. I told God recently, I said Lord I give you my word that I will not fear, I will not entertain fear. Fear has stolen so much from me so I had to promise God strongly that I will not fear, rather I will trust Him knowing that He will not fail me. Now if I make God a promise and do not keep it, how will I expect God to confirm His word to me? That is how I hold myself accountable were fear is concerned since it has an eternal consequence. You should do the same.

What has He said to you personally over time?

The personal revelation that you have received over time will become your bailout in time of adversity. Many times, I tell you I have had to stand my ground simply based on what the Holy Spirit delivered to me when I had a need. Many years ago, I was under a lot of pressure and I was so weighed down and I experienced a heart condition. I was in service one morning and I heard the Holy spirit say within me concerning that condition as my mind began to be troubled, He said "you have a Divine nature" at that time I had no clue where that Scripture was in the Bible but when your word comes, it settles every conflict. That is exactly what I experienced, every conflict in my heart was settled, comfort came and peace came and that thing disappear when I was not looking.

What has He said to you. That became my word in season. If the enemy threatens, I can take that word again, the Lord will remind me and it has the exact same effect in any other situation as it did the first time. I later found that Scripture in 2 Peter 1: 1- 4

Just to mention a few, the Lord has said to me as I used a product that I found out was toxic and I was about to say – these things can kill- and He intercepted my thoughts before they formed into words and said "nothing can Kill you" that is according to our authority as a believer which says "and these signs shall follow those that believe, in my name if they take up any deadly thing it shall not harm them and that has also became listed as my Word in season.

Keep a list of those promises that the Lord has said to you one time or the other and keep them in front of you where you can see them easily and they will answer for you in time of need.

Many years ago, I had a dream that I was afflicted with disease and I woke up greatly distressed and as I cried out to the Lord and I Heard him say clearly "it would have been so but Jesus Christ the Son of the Living God loved you and gave Himself for you" again that settled every conflict and I was at peace. Then later He said that word applies to every negative suggestion that the enemy may bring up. That word is not only for me, it is for everyone I share it with. But then again it is your own word and for me it is my word in season.

At any time earnestly expect the Lord to send you His word for your breakthrough deliverance and turn around, they are all deposited in His word for us. So, look to the Word for your deliverance healing and breakthrough today. He will send you;

Your sent word
Your now word
Your word in season
Your right word

I said that fear has an eternal consequence. In Revelation Chapter 21 I saw this truth and that day, it put fear in its place in my life. This is what the scripture says about fear.

But the fearful, and unbelieving, and the abominable, and murderers, and whoremongers, and sorcerers, and idolaters, and all liars, shall have their part in the lake which burn with fire and brimstone: which is the second death. Revelation "21: 8

Notice that unbelief and doubt produce fear. That is the source of fear right there so you will know how to identify it. Fear also comes from lack of hearing and continuing to hear the word of God. If you have starved your spirit-man, then fear will reign in your heart because the basic ingredient that produces and supplies faith which is the Word of God is absent.

I choose to believe God any way, things may not look like it will change, it may be as hopeless as can be, but I believe God anyway, He is the solution carrier, in Him is the way out of any kind of trouble, He said He will be with you, why? He will deliver you and set you far above that thing that is threatening you. That is great confidence for me.

I must believe Him on purpose even when I do not feel like it and would rather worry, feel sorry for myself or panic and fear, rather I switch to trust mode and become quiet trusting and I keep my eye on the Word and keep the Word in my ear to build my faith. Notice that it is a conscious effort not a passive thing that we do to try God and see if it will work, we do not try faith, if you do that you will fail. Faith is backed up by the word of God, what God has said, therefore it CANNOT FAIL you.

We must train our hearts to believe God on purpose especially in the days that we now live in. In the last days, perilous times will come. Jesus said that "men's heart will fail for fear" so it is for your own benefit that you train not to entertain fear, the guarantee is that God has said "I am your shield" therefore anything that comes to you must come through Him. Anything He allows to come He has equipped you to overcome it because He is with you in the first place.

Why you must not fear? You will hear and see things in this last days that your ears will tingle. But you must not fear. The enemy may threaten you or your family but you must not fear. You must trust and rest.

Fear leads to Error

The first thing that presents its self in a crisis is fear, you cannot control what tries to come upon you, it is your response that counts. Kenneth E Hagin says "you cannot prevent a bird from flying over your head but you can prevent it from perching on your head and building a nest there" think about that. Panic will produce fear if you do not turn on the switch of faith straight away.

Do nothing out of fear, He that believes does not make haste.

Listen for His voice or go straight to the word or listen to a message. Expose yourself to the word, you will certainly hear Him either through the message you are hearing or that message will clear the way for your spirit man to take charge and lead you out by the prompting of the Holy Spirit.

Now it is your faith that will overcome the world and its systems, so you must build your faith on purpose against the day of adversity! Keep hearing and hearing the Word sustain your time and place of fellowship. Spend time in the word and in prayer. We have been instructed to pray without ceasing, and we ought always to pray and not to faint. Pray also that you do not enter into temptation Jesus told us. Prayer gives you a confidence to confront the affairs of life. Prayer gives us a confidence that God is with us. Prayer sustains divine presence in your life. Pray always.

You must build a relationship with the Holy Spirit. He is God with us. Train to be conscious of His divine presence as our Comforter. He is the one sent to walk alongside us to fulfil the counsel of God and to lead us into fulfilling our God ordained destiny. Get to know Him learn all you can about Him. And after you have done all:

Take a stand of faith

Decide that you will rather believe God and put all your faith and trust in Him and in His word. He has never failed

God will honour your faith

God will certainly honour your faith in Him.

The Word of God will not fail you

I often picture our Lord Jesus walking on water as the word of God walking on water. He is the word of God made flesh. He walked on water and did not sink so have this picture in your heart and mind that in the same way you and I can stand on the word of God in the area of our need and have the full assurance and confidence that it will not fail. We will not sink.

If you are standing on the Word, then that situation must be able to sink the Word of God which is God to be able to sink you. Think on that.

9

Do not forsake your Mercy

They that observe lying vanities forsake their own
mercy. Jonah 2:8

After many years of always running to God in fear
that came from challenges, I became conscious of
the fact that my relationship with God was based
on my fear of what the enemy can do in my life. At the instance of any kind of symptom in my body, I would run to
God not in faith but in fear. One day I asked the Lord sin-
cerely how did I get to this place of fear and His immediate
response was – you have believed a lie.

That statement of truth struck me, I was not in any way
expecting that response. I thought on this for a while and
the next thing to do was that the solution to this was that I
must consciously begin to believe the word of God no
matter what I felt or saw. The Lord said to me "Ema answer every lie with the truth, refuse to believe a lie" For

instance, when the thought comes to you that you will never recover from a condition, you know that it is a lie. Why? Because the Word which is truth says that "with His stripes we are healed" Why? Because our sins are forgiven us, therefore, sickness and disease cannot prevail against us. There is so much more in our arsenal of truth to use and counter every lie that presents itself.

If the thought that – God will not do anything about that situation because you have not been completely faithful to Him. Then that is a lie, because the Scripture says that – He will not treat us as our sins deserve, like as a Father pities His children so that Lord has mercy upon them that fear Him. Psalm 103 as our focus in this book says – He was wounded for our transgression, bruised for our iniquity and the chastisement of our peace was upon Him and with His stripes, we are healed Isaiah 53: 5 - Our sins are forgiven us.

Who shall lay anything to the charge of God's elect? It is God that justifies. 34 Who is he that condemns? It is Christ that died, yea rather, that is risen again, who is even at the right hand of God, who also makes intercession for us. Romans 8: 33 - 34

If the thought that God does not care about you comes, well you can replace that with this amazing truth that says, "if He [God] did not spare his own Son but gave Him up to die for us, will he not with the gift of His Son freely give us all things?" this is a question, think about it and answer it for yourself.

It is also said that, if we believe not, yet he abides faithful: He cannot deny himself" - 2 Timothy 2:13 so if you are pushed to the place where you begin to wonder if things will change and doubts begins to come, God is constant, He is not at this point affected by your doubt. He remains faithful because that is who He is. And that is why we can trust, depend on Him in the face of contrary circumstances.

There is mercy in our God

Our Scripture focus for this chapter Jonah 3: 8 says that "if we observe lying vanities, we forsake our mercy" What does this mean?

Things are not always the way that they appear to be. Many times, the things that we panic about and become alarmed and anxious are just lying vanities. Our minds blow them out of proportion. We are to renew our mind and bring it under the complete control of the Word of God or it will rob us of our mercy.

The Prophet calls it "lying vanity" He is saying that, that situation is not as bad as it seems or looks if we can dare to believe God. I will put it this way, the only doubt that you are allowed to have, is to doubt your own doubt and doubt the suggestions of your mind and chose consciously to believe God instead. Hope against hope and believe God anyway, that what He has promised, He is not only able to perform but that He is willing to perform it if we will believe Him for it.

There is always mercy in God. He offered that we come to "the throne of Grace with Boldness and obtain Mercy" stop there just yet. The word obtain there means to "take" or collect mercy. In this place of the throne of Grace, mercy is handed out to us. In this place, every judgment is suspended, it is called the throne of Grace. God Himself assumes responsibility for all your mistakes and short comings. He declares you – not guilty – that is the only way that you can have mercy, and mercy is handed out to you so that you can overcome that situation. Here God over rules all charges brought against you. Glory to God forever!

Your healing and deliverance is handed out to you free of charge because it has already been paid for. You must reach out and collect it – you must take it by faith. That is why the Prophet says that - if you make the reality or facts which he calls "lying vanities" – [a thing that does not have any roots or foundation. It is founded on lies and deception] of that condition your focus, you will forsake the mercy that has already been provided and reserved – made available for you. Think about that.

Now in this same place, it says that we can locate – find Grace to help us in our time of need. One translation says, "necessary help" that is the specific help that you need is made available to you at your request. If you need the Grace of healing to help in this time of need, He says, come and you will find it here. If it is the Grace for finance or economic bailout, He said you can locate it here and it is yours. Why is it that you have need of? There is an open invitation for us to come, not fearful and timid, but with boldness and full assurance of faith that God will not lie and His word will not fail. He does not condemn us.

He has said – come to the throne of Grace, with boldness and obtain mercy and find Grace to help in this time of need!

Bring Repentance

Now 1 John 1: 9 says: *8 If we say that we have no sin, we deceive ourselves, and the truth is not in us. 9 If we confess our sins, he is faithful and just to forgive us our sins, and to cleanse us from all unrighteousness. 10 If we say that we have not sinned, we make him a liar, and his word is not in us.* The word of God is very clear. We must be quick to bring repentance before God for any act of unrighteousness. What we know of or what we do not know of. We can ask the Lord to show us areas in our lives that we need to clean up. Whatever the Holy spirit has quickened in us as not pleasing to God, we must be quick to repents and bring it under that Cross of Calvary. Recently I had to ask the Lord to search my heart to see if there be any evil way or any evil heart of unbelief in me so that I can repent of it.

God Himself will cleanse us from all unrighteousness. We must not remain in the place of guilt and condemnation before God. He says to me "Ema, I do not condemn you' that gives me confidence before God always. We are to wear His righteousness as a garment so that the enemy will not gain any occasion against us.

Your Word in season
THE LORD OUR HELP
For the Lord GOD will help me; therefore, shall I not be confounded: therefore, have I set my face like a flint, and I know that I shall not be ashamed. 8 He is near that justifies me; who will contend with me? let us stand together: who is mine adversary? let him come near to me. 9 Behold, the Lord GOD will help me; who is he that shall condemn me? lo, they all shall wax old as a garment; the moth shall eat them up. Isaiah 50: 7 – 9

10

Take your stand of faith in the word of God

Jesus has paid a high price for us to go free – So take a stand of faith
Jesus said, "Believe and doubt not"
Jesus said, "Speak to the mountain; it should obey you"

Declare that you may be Justified
Isa 43: 26

What I want you to do in this section is that you record with your own voice any section of this book that really speaks to you on any portable device like your phone, a tablet or even a recorder. Listen to it repeatedly until it begins to speak to you. What this will do is that you can hear the truth out of your own mouth. When you tell yourself the truth it is a lot easier to persuade your heart to believe.

Our ability to receive from God absolutely depends on our ability to believe Him, "for as many as believed on Him, to them gave He power to become the sons of God" John 1: 12 and it is also written "I am the LORD thy God, which brought thee out of the land of Egypt: open thy mouth wide, and I will fill it." Psalms 81:10

When you believe in Jesus, you activate the power to become what you believe. Now it is worth doing whatever it takes to persuade our heart to believe God were our healing or breakthrough or deliverance of any kind is concerned.

Our Father Abraham had this testimony;

"(As it is written, I have made thee a father of many nations) before him whom he believed, even God, who quickens the dead, and calls those things which be not as though they were. 18 Who against hope believed in hope, that he might become the father of many nations, according to that which was spoken, so shall thy seed be. 19 And being not weak in faith, he considered not his own body now dead, when he was about an hundred years old, neither yet the deadness of Sara's womb: 20 He staggered not at the promise of God through unbelief; but was strong in faith, giving glory to God; 21 And being fully persuaded that, what he had promised, he was able also to perform. 22 And therefore it was imputed to him for righteousness"

Now within the context of this book right now, I want you to put yourself and whatever situation that you have believed God for in this portion of Scripture. Now if you desire healing it reads like this;

(As it is written, with His stripes, you were healed) before him whom I believe, even God, who quickens the dead, and calls those things which be not as though they were. Who against hope I believe in hope, that I might become completely healed and work in divine health now, according to that which was spoken, Himself took our infirmities and bore our sicknesses. And being not weak in faith, I consider not my own body now weak or in pain, or the reports of the Physicians: I stagger not at the promise of God through unbelief; but I am strong in faith, giving glory to God; **And being fully persuaded that, what he has promised, He is able also to perform**. 22 And therefore it is imputed to me for righteousness. [My right to become and experience everything that God has promised me]

Now open your heart, meditate on this day and night and it will fully persuade your heart to believe and in the same way that Our father Abraham obtained the promise, so will you be completely healed and divine health will become your testimony and you will become a blessing to many through your own testimony. So, you see that God is not so much focused on you being healed and totally set free but He is looking at the bigger picture. It is always "I will bless you and make you a blessing" I will heal you and make you a healer "blessing" I will deliver you and make you a deliverer, as so forth.

You see that it means a lot to God that you and I be healed and delivered so that we can bring the same blessing to many. God can then spread the Blessing through us to the rest of mankind. The Scripture puts it this way, it says:

> Blessed be God, even the Father of our Lord Je-
> sus Christ, the Father of mercies, and the God of
> all comfort; 4 Who comforts us in all our tribula-
> tion, that we may be able to comfort them which
> are in any trouble, by the comfort wherewith we
> ourselves are comforted of God. 2 Corinthians 1:
> 3 – 4

Whatever you are desiring from God today, see the bigger picture. Let God show you how much of a blessing it
would be for you to be healed than for that condition to be
prolong in your life. Think about this, if you were God,
what would you rather have, if you had the ability to do for
your children what they desire, which one would you do?
Which one will be a greater witness to your faithfulness
and kindness? Which one will attract many to you? What
would you rather do?

I am sure you would rather, your children be delivered
and made free so that the world may see your goodness
and be attracted to you. Trust God in this way and have
faith in Him, take him at His word, become fully persuaded
that what He has promised, he is also able to perform it for
you especially when He has paid such a high price to do
this for you in sending His only begotten son to die such a
brutal death. God wants you well and He has paid the price
for it, so believe Him today and go ahead and receive [take,
collect] your healing, deliverance or breakthrough today.
Hallelujah!

He is our Peace

I was saying to my children recently that the single most
important thing for us is peace. When God wants to bless a

people, he gives them rest round about. When you have peace, you are progressive and it is easy for you to become prosperous and fruitful. The right conditions surround you and opportunities are attracted to you. A tranquil life naturally promotes the Blessing. What are we talking about here?

In Isaiah 53 verse 4 it is written that "the chastisement – punishment – penalty – cost – of our peace was put upon Jesus and with His stripes we are healed.

I went ahead to look more closely to these things. Jesus in responding to the faith of the four friends that tore that roof so that they could lower their friend down to Jesus, He said to the sick man "your sins are forgiven you" why did he say that? After all the man was not caught doing anything wrong at the time neither was Jesus referring to their act of destroying another man's property just to get to Him as sin. He saw what the friends did, the effort they made to bring their sick friend to Jesus as an act of their faith, it is said "and Jesus seeing their faith" so what was He talking about here as He said your sins are forgiven, take up your bed and go home?

Jesus was dealing with the root of sicknesses and disease, there is no point in cutting a tree from the stalk, it will grow again from the root. Jesus attacked that thing from the root. If you look at that portion of Scripture, it deals with the root of infirmity which is the source of sickness and disease of any kind. The nature of sin that brought sickness and disease into humanity.

In verse 4 of Isaiah 53 It is said "Surely, he hath borne our griefs, and carried our sorrows" Matthew 8: 17 in referencing this Scripture puts it this way "Himself took our infirmities and bore our sicknesses" and 1Peter 2: 24 says; "Who His own self bore our sins in His body on the tree"

Everything that sin brought upon humanity, Jesus took in His own body. He became sin. He became sin for us who knew no sin, so that you and I may become the righteousness of God through Him. Think about that for a moment. In dealing with sin, everything else that proceeds from sin is completely dealt with.

When you wake up to the reality of what Salvation has brought for you and as faith comes through this knowledge, every lie must submit to the truth. No mater by what name that condition is named, when light comes such as this one, that darkness in form of sickness and disease must disperse. And let me tell you this, when light comes darkness leaves instantly.

That is why when Jesus healed, it was always said "and immediately" You see it is at the instance of revelation that deliverance comes, it does not matter if the symptoms persist, I tell you the truth, the foundation of that condition in your life has been completely removed and destroyed, it no longer exist to feed and support its growth so it must die now. Remember the fig tree!

The price of our Peace has been fully paid

But he was wounded for our transgressions; he was bruised for our iniquities: the chastisement of our peace was upon him; and with his stripes we are healed. Isa 53: 5

God went ahead through the death of His Son Jesus to pay the price to bring us into a covenant of peace. I decided to make Isaiah 53: 4 and 5 my foundation Scripture for life until I see Messiah face to face. Why is that? because looking closely and as the Holy Spirit opens the eye of my understanding, I have come to see that it holds the key to everything that I will ever need not only in this life but for eternity. This is where everything was settled for me.

This is where all the price was fully borne for my total liberty to live the good life. Here, we see sin the mother of all evil dealt with. As we saw earlier, if you want to eradicate anything, go to the root and it is gone. So here I see and keep it in front of me that my sins have been forgiven not only my mistakes and error and all my short comings and poor choices, but the very nature of sin itself, the very thing that made me subject to the law of sin and death which produces all evil like sickness disease, poverty lack want and every evil work.

The very desire to do wrong the lean towards compromise. That nature of sin no longer operates within me. Now another law is working within me and that is the Law of the spirit of life in Christ Jesus. This law is powered by the Grace of God through righteousness unto eternal life by Jesus Christ our Lord. Glory to God forever!

With sin out of the way, the price is paid for our peace, that tranquil life that Adam once had in the Garden was once again restored to us through the sacrifice of our Lord Jesus Christ. Mind you all of this is only possible by our ability to simply take God at His word and persuade our heart to believe. At this point I want you to carefully look at the full implication of the word peace that Jesus paid the price to bring to us.

You will Live – For He is your Peace

Interestingly, when Gideon saw the angel of the Lord and became afraid believing that He most certainly was going to die, because it was said and it was the truth that you see God and die. This incident is where God revealed

Himself as JEHOVAH SHALOM the LORD OUR PEACE.

The Angel said to Him, "you shall not die" and the Lord Jesus Himself is saying to you today "I have come that you may have life and that you may have it more abundantly" because the mission of the Lord must surely be fulfilled in your life. Jesus has paid a high price for you to live. He gave his life to sickness and disease, His gave His life to death so that you may live. He took your place in sickness and disease, He took your place in death and He is saying to you today, LIVE!

And the LORD said unto him, Peace be unto thee; fear not: thou shalt not die. 24 Then Gideon built an altar there unto the LORD, and called it Jehovah shalom: The Lord your Peace Judges 6: 23 – 24. The word Shalom here means exactly the same as the word "peace" found in Isaiah 53: 5 – which says that "the chastisement of our peace was upon Him" Meaning that - the punishment required to purchase our Shalom – or to bring us into the Covenant of Peace was upon Jesus.

Shalom: Covenant of Peace
Definition: **To be in a covenant of peace, be at peace**
- to be at peace
- peaceful one (participle)
- one in covenant of peace (participle)
- to make peace with
- to cause to be at peace
- to live in peace
- to be complete, be sound
- to be complete, be finished, be ended

- to be sound, be uninjured
- to complete, finish
- to make safe
- to make whole or good, restore, make compensation
- to make good, pay
- to requite, recompense, reward
- to be performed
- to be repaid, be requited
- to complete, perform
- to make an end of

King James Word Usage - Total: 116

To pay- peace - recompense - reward - render - restore - repay - perform - good - end - requite - restitution - finished - again - amends - full

The Word Peace used in Isaiah 53: 5 is translated to mean the following:

completeness, soundness, welfare, peace

completeness (in number)

safety, soundness (in body)

welfare, health, prosperity

peace, quiet, tranquility, contentment

peace, friendship

of human relationships

with God, especially in covenant relationship

peace (from war)

peace (as adjective)

Meditate on this. This is what Jesus died to paid the price for you and me.

11

Our Declaration of faith

I made a recording with this revelation declaring over myself and my entire family everything that the peace Jesus paid the price for has brought to us and I want you to go ahead now, make the effort, record this in your own voice no matter how weak you are, the very process of doing this will provoke the virtue [power] in this truth and healing will begin to saturate your entire system and as you keep listening complete deliverance will come to you. Now do it don't put it off, just do it.

Record this with your own voice: This is all based on Isaiah 53: 5 - This recording will be approximately 20 mins.

Father in the name of Jesus, I declare the covenant of peace in my life and family right now and this translates to my total health and my peace. For the punishment that brought us into the Covenant of wealth, Covenant of peace, that peace O Lord God that was spoken to Gideon in Judges chapter 6 verse 24, it said "peace unto you, you will not die, peace to you, do not fear, you shall not die" Lord you said to Gideon, peace to you, do not fear, you shall not die. This peace is the Covenant of peace coming from Jesus – The Lord our Peace – JEHOVAH SHA-LOM. He is my peace.

In the name of our Lord Jesus Christ, In Isaiah 54 verse 10 it is also written "the mountains shall depart and the hills be removed but my kindness shall not depart from you neither shall the Covenant of my peace be removed said the Lord that has had mercy on you. *[Say this again. Pray in the spirit in between as you are making this declaration so that revelation will come to you – it will open to you]*

Brief interlude
God Promises the Covenant of Peace
This is the Word of the Lord: "the silver is mine the Gold is mine, says the Lord Almighty, the Glory of this present house is greater that the glory of the former house said the Lord Almighty and in this place, I have granted peace, in this place I have given peace in the mighty name of our Lord Jesus Christ. Pause and pray in the spirit at this point.

This Covenant of peace is also established in the book of Ezekiel and it says: And I will make with them a covenant of peace, and will cause the evil beasts to cease out of the land: and they shall dwell safely in the wilderness, and sleep in the woods. Ezekiel 34: 25

And again, it is written; Moreover, I will make a covenant of peace with them; it shall be an everlasting covenant with them: and I will place them, and multiply them, and will set my sanctuary in the midst of them for evermore. Ezekiel 37:26

Now continue with your recording

Father you brought the Covenant of your peace and established it in my life in Christ Jesus, you have brought me into the Covenant of peace through Christ Jesus. You are the LORD MY PEACE – JEHOVAH SHALOM – The Lord my peace; meaning the Lord my completeness, because the punishment required to establish my completeness, the chastisement of my peace, the punishment required to bring me into completeness, soundness welfare, peace, completeness in number; meaning that I will not lose anything [my children] no member of my family will be lost. In the name of our Lord Jesus Christ. We will have no losses spiritually, physically in the name of Jesus.

My family is intact. I have safety, meaning no accidents, we have preservation and covering. I have soundness in my body in the name of Jesus Christ, nothing missing nothing broken, physical health, soundness in my children, welfare with the full meaning of it which is: exemption from calamity, want and lack and I have prosperity. In the name of our Lord Jesus Christ.

I have welfare as we know it, divine health; in the name of our Lord Jesus Christ. Mental health, physical health, financial health, spiritual health, health in my relationships. In the name of our Lord Jesus Christ. I have Prosperity and Peace, quietness, a re-enforcement of peace, which is perfect peace. Tranquility, a tranquil state of affairs, I am unruffled. I have contentment, I am supplied, library supplied lacking nothing.

I have Peace and friendship of human relationships, relationship with God especially in Covenant. Peace from any kind of war. Meaning that my territory has rest round about. I have all round rest. I have active peace – I have peace that I can experience actively, peace you can touch, peace you can feel, in the name of our Lord Jesus Christ. Noticeable peace, not peace that one is looking for, noticeable peace.

This Covenant of peace brings me health and peace it makes me peaceful, I am peaceful, I have prosperity and safety. They will salute me – I have favour with man.

Welfare – I am in a state of wellbeing, so the punishment required for my wellbeing and our wellbeing as a family has been paid for. I have ease, I am favourable and I have friendship. I will be greeted by men; I am favoured. I have Divine health. I have Perfect peace, I am peaceful. I have Prosperity.

Rose: I have beauty

I have safety – I am secure – I have trust and welfare, I am in a state of wellbeing. I am at peace, I am holy, all is well with me. Everything is alright. I am peaceful. I have shalom. I am favourable. This is for me a time of peace; I am at peace. In the name of Jesus Christ. I have harmony – there is order in my life, everything is in order in my life. I am peaceful. I enjoy productivity in the name of our Lord Jesus Christ, I am productive.

I have success taken completely, the assurance of prosperity, welfare and the wellbeing. In the name of our Lord Jesus Christ.

We sow in peace – I escape this condition unscathed, I have welfare and wellbeing. We have prosperity and all round rest. Rest from war – resulting in all round rest.

To crown it all Lord – I am be at Peace, in a Covenant of Peace.

The Punishment that was laid upon Jesus, the punishment that was required to bring me into a Covenant of peace, that punishment to cause me to be at peace, to be a peaceful one, one in Covenant of Peace, to make peace with, to cause me to be at peace, that is all round rest, to live in peace, to be complete, to be sound, Jesus Christ paid the price for.

The punishment for me to be complete, to be finished, to be ended, everything concerning me, concerning my children, concerning my family has been completed, and we have now been put in the middle of this completeness to live it. We are living a completed life; our life is finished we are living in a finished work.

For we are recreated in Christ Jesus unto good works taking paths that the Lord has pre-arranged and made ready for us. I am living the good life that the Lord has made ready for me. A readymade life. I am sound. I am injured. I am complete, finished, make sound and safe and to make whole and good. Restore and make compensation. To make good and to pay in the name of Jesus Christ.

To requite me to recompense me, the punishment and the price for me to be requited, the price for my recompense my reward was put upon Jesus. I am to be performed because the price for the plan of God for me to be performed has been paid for – I am to be repaid – by an over payment – the performance of those things that were told me of the Lord. They shall be a performance of everything that has been told me of the Lord.

To complete, perform and to make an end of. To make an end of feebleness in my life. Finally, to make an end of feebleness – spirit of feebleness Jesus Christ has paid the price for you to end in my life.

Lack and want Jesus Christ paid the price for you to end in my life. He paid the price for my sin and my short comings and all my mistakes and poor choices. I declare the righteousness of Jesus Christ because my sins are forgiven me, In the name of our Lord Jesus Christ.

The price for an end to sickness and infirmity has been fully paid for – and I take it – I take it now – In the name of our Lord Jesus Christ. I live the good life – that finished work because the price for it to be performed in my life has been fully paid for. Therefore, I take it, for it is mine. In the name of our Lord Jesus Christ. [pause and pray in the spirit]

Holy Communion

Therefore, Lord I take this Holy Communion and I seal the Word of God in my life and declare peace – all round rest – peace in every area of my life – peace across our Family – peace in the life of the children – In the mighty name of our Lord Jesus Christ. I will not eat of this table unworthily for my sins are forgiven me – I receive this table as a Covenant and as a testimony – as a seal of the Covenant of peace – I take my healing and I take my deliverance now, so that it may be fulfilled in my life that which was spoken by Isaiah the prophet saying

I declare that I am at peace in the name of our Lord Jesus Christ – wealth and riches are in my house – I will not forget prosperity – I will not leave prosperity on the table - I am prosperous – Holy Ghost – In the name of our Lord

Jesus Christ – I partner with you to make wealth in the name of our Lord Jesus Christ. And Father to you alone be all the Glory.

Lord as I eat of your flesh – I am made whole and sound and perfect - and I take all the virtues of Jesus – the spirit of wisdom and Understanding, and the spirit of meekness - for in Him are hidden all the treasures of wisdom ad knowledge and we are complete I Him – I provoke wisdom by this table of the Covenant – I provoke the power in the name of our Lord Jesus Christ.

Jesus Christ the wisdom of God and the power of God – **as I eat of your flesh** – I provoke that spirit of wisdom – the Bible says that you always know what to do – that I will know what to do always – I have understanding – clarity of vision – clarity of my assignment in the name of our Lord Jesus Christ

Supernatural supply and abundance: - Jesus in your body [the bread] are houses – cars – anything that I so desire – and I take it all in the name of Jesus Christ our Lord.

By the cup – I receive the forgiveness of sins across my family network – in the mighty miraculous name of Jesus Christ our Lord – I receive the life of Jesus – I declare that eternal life is working in me – immortality is working in me swallowing up mortality – I receive healing and health – I receive life in my cells – life in all my organs – from the crown of my head to the soles of my feet

I receive life – I take healing – I take deliverance in the name of our Lord Jesus Christ – and by the Blood of Jesus – the works of the devil are all destroyed in my life and family – and destroyed in my body – for my body is the temple of the Holy Spirit – therefore – Lord I glorify you in my body and in my spirit which belongs to you – for I have been bought with a price – the token of my redemption is the precious blood of Jesus –

Therefore what so ever my heavenly Father has not planted in my body – I command you this day – be rooted up and be cast into the lake of fire – in the name of our Lord Jesus Christ – Father I give you thanks -   I receive the very life of Jesus at this Holy Communion Table – I declare that I am one with you – I live by you – I live like you – and I am one with you – and I live and not die – and if you tarry – you will raise me up at the last day – Lord thank you for length of days – for it is written that you satisfy me with long life and show me your Salvation –

Thank you Lord God of Heaven – thank you for the Covenant of peace – I worship you the Lord my Peace – You are the Lord the Lord my Peace – Lord pass to and fro across our family network – in the midst of the children – the Lord the Lord – our peace – I worship you mighty God - pass through this home, pass through us O Lord God and let your Goodness pass before us – I declare the peace of all my children for they are taught of you Lord and great is their peace. We return all the glory to you Lord – In Jesus name Amen.

This is the full declaration; you can adopt and change it to your own particular need. Be blessed!

12

Having done all to stand – Stand

Fight the good fight of faith

Having done all, we are instructed to stand our ground. Everything must submit to the counsel of the word of God. Sometimes this is when our faith comes under severe attack. Faith can be tried and will be also. How do we keep doubt and unbelief out during the time between when we release our faith and when we see the manifestation of what we desire?

We keep the word of God in our eye and our ear streaming through into our heart and coming out of our mouth. As we continue to do this we are feeding our faith and keeping our faith strong. I heard Gloria Copeland say that in the early days of her Christian life – she was not getting results and she inquired of the Lord and the word of the Lord came to her that "In consistency – lies the power" think about that for a moment. You must continue to do what you have been doing.

Ask in prayer to see if there is something that you are missing and if not then be consistent in what you know to do. If there is anything else, God is faithful to bring that information to you. Kenneth E Hagin said, "walk in the light you already have" Do what you already know to do. Have faith in God put your trust in Him – believe the Word and it will not fail you. Remember that Jesus walked on water. I see that as the word of God walking on water and it did not sink. Stay with the Word we have steadily come to the days of the manifestation of God's Grace as never before- so believe God and Healing always comes.

Do not cast away your confidence

The Word of God says this "Let us hold fast the profession of our faith without wavering; (for he is faithful that promised;)"

Cast not away therefore your confidence, which hath great recompense of reward. 36 For ye have need of patience, that, after ye have done the will of God, ye might receive the promise. 37 For yet a little while, and he that shall come will come, and will not tarry. 38 Now the just shall live by faith: but if any man draw back, my soul shall have no pleasure in him. 39 But we are not of them who draw back unto perdition; but of them that believe to the saving of the soul. Hebrews 10: 23 / 35 -39

It will speak, and the result will surely come

You are encouraged to hold onto your faith in the full assurance that the result that you desire of God will surely come and not delay. Of course this is talking about the coming of the Messiah- but God is speaking to you and me also as we stand in faith for our healing – deliverance of any kind or breakthrough that we desire of God- the same instruction applies – Hold fast to the profession [confession] of your faith without wavering" Jesus said in Mark 11: 23 "believe and doubt not in your heart" and He also said "fear not believe only" so you and I have a full assurance of faith that what we believe God for will surely come.

Remember Hannah- after she believed the word of the Prophet of God– she went her way and her countenance was no longer sad. This is how you hold onto your faith- Jesus is saying to you now – "go your way – meaning – Go about your business – what you have believed for will be done for you as you have believed. This is where we stand in our faith to receive.

You exercise your faith by going about your business – you go about doing those things that you put on hold because of that condition or situation– all the while keeping the word of God in front of you and in your ear. Remember that at this time the faith of Jesus has been activated, for "He ever lives to make intercession for us who have come to the Father through Him" Hebrews 7: 25 And His faith and prayer is working for you right now to deliver your desired result. Hallelujah!

Take your Healing now

We were praying recently on our prayer forum for healing and the Lord had given me this Scripture and I was meditating on it and I saw that the Word saved is translated to also mean – heal – or healing – think about that. For by

Grace are you saved through faith; and that not of your-selves: it is the gift of God: Ephesians 2: 8 What this is saying to us is that- every promise of God to us – all our inheritance - everything that we will ever desire of God – has been given by Grace through faith as a gift of God.

A few years ago, I had not received this scripture by rev-elation and I was crying out to God to heal me of weakness and a state of un-wellnesses. Two major things happened during this time.

I kept listening and listening to the word of God to build my faith but I struggled to believe – I did not doubt but at the same time I was still trying to understand how faith works so that I can be healed. One day – I suppose I was quiet enough for the Lord to get a word in – you see in our quest to make God do what we want- we keep talking and talking and crying and we become overwhelmed by our emotions so much so that we keep God out or we cannot hear Him as He brings us that word of Comfort and healing.

Healing comes by the Word of God that comes by reve-lation and, by the Word that we simply receive by faith. Think about that. Now the Lord said to me "it is not your faith that will heal you- you are healed by my Grace" that stopped me in my tracks. The Grace of God as my source of healing has never been taught me – or I have never heard that my healing comes by the Grace of God through my faith. I can't make God heal me, He has already healed me by Grace and I receive it through faith as a gift of God.

So, I cannot now boast that my faith made God to heal me our do anything He has already finished in redemption. That word brought instant relieve and faith grew in my heart and every pressure to make God heal me disappeared and I rested and thought on that word and healing came.

Again, as I thought on why I was so fearful I decided on purpose that I will no longer run to God in fear every time I feel something in my body – because that is what the enemy wants. I will not be driven by fear – rather I will go to God in faith and I will trust and rest. The Lord said to me that the reason I had prolonged condition in my body was because – hear this – "you have believed a lie" shocked again- and since I have made a conscious effort to do two things

- I will not fear
- I will believe the word of God when my mind suggests anything that will bring fear- I cast it down and chose to believe the Word of God instead.
- I say, "I will trust and not fear"

I pray that this blesses you. The Lord had said to me that I should answer every lie with the truth. Now as we mediate on this Scripture it is telling us that we are Saved, also meaning that we are Healed – delivered, kept safe and sound from danger or destruction – saved from disease – made well – restored to health – and rescued all of this by the Grace of God through faith. Our faith does not make it happen – it has already been done – Grace has done it – our faith brings it to us as a gift of God – it goes on to say it is so that no man should boast – you cannot say it is my ability to do so and so that brought me healing – no, your healing and mine is by the Grace of God – through our faith – that is as we believe and receive it. We take it and make it ours.

I said in that prayer meeting that a gift – we do not work for – many times we do not deserve some gifts that we receive, in that case, it comes as a favour and simply an act of love from the giver of that gift to us. – even if we should deserve this kind of Gift – Jesus paid the price that brought us into favour with God to warrant this gift – so what should we do with any gift – well we go ahead and receive it – we take it and begin to enjoy it. That Scripture spells it out for us clearly so receive it – take your healing – deliverance – breakthrough or anything you desire of God as a gift that has come as a Grace of God through your faith. Glory to God!

Definition the Word "Saved"

To save, keep safe and sound, to rescue from danger or destruction

One (from injury or peril)

To save a suffering one (from perishing), i.e. one suffering from disease, to make well, heal, restore to health

To preserve one who is in danger of destruction, to save or rescue

To save in the technical biblical sense

To deliver from the penalties of the Messianic judgment 1b

To save from the evils which obstruct the reception of the Messianic deliverance

A Word in Season
IT IS FINISHED
"our Healing has been finished, it if a gift of God by Grace. We take it now and begin to eat the fruit of our healing"
Finally, my brethren think on this - meditate on these things and persuade your heart to fully believe and enjoy

what the Grace of God has given us. Say this: I choose to believe God – and say like Apostle Paul said in the face of death and destruction – I believe God - that it will be even as it has been told me of the Lord – Peace!

"You have received Jesus as your Savior- now receive Him as your Healer – the author and finisher of our faith"

13

The Joy of the Lord is your strength

Joy is not an emotion of the flesh it is a fruit of the spirit and joy is not a result of what is happening around us, with us and to us, Joy is a supernatural force that carries the power of God and it works by faith. We activate Joy by faith and put it to work for us. Three Scriptures tell us the importance of the force of Joy to the believer.

Nehemiah 8: 10 says, "the Joy of the Lord is your strength" in the face of challenges and great difficulty and strong opposition, he sent that message to Israel. So, we draw strength from the force of Joy to confront any challenge and any opposition in life. Now we see in Isaiah 12: 3, it says:

"Joyful thanksgiving of the faithful for the mercies of God"

And in that day [which is today – Now] you shall say, O LORD, I will praise you: though you were angry with me, your anger is turned away, and you comforted me. 2 Behold, God is my salvation; I will trust, and not be afraid: for the LORD JEHOVAH is my strength and my song; he also is become my salvation. 3 **Therefore with joy shall you draw water out of the wells of salvation.**

This your testimony and the fruit and result of the force of Joy

4 And in that day, shall you say, Praise the LORD, call upon his name, declare his doings among the people, make mention that his name is exalted. 5 Sing unto the LORD; for he has done excellent things: this is known in all the earth. 6 Cry out and shout, you inhabitant of Zion: for great is the Holy One of Israel in the midst of you.

Meditate on that, this is your testimony right there. Take it and believe it and rejoice! With Joy, we draw from the wells of Salvation. Joy is the bucket that we use to lower down into the rich treasury of Salvation to draw anything that we need. And it is not an act of the will, it is an act of faith, you do not have to feel like it, nothing will motivate it, in most cases everything around you are contrary to it, but it is the single most potent source and connection to our inheritance in redemption. Joy connects you to your healing and deliverance. You activate it by faith.

With Joy, you draw healing and heal from the wells of Salvation. Glory to God forever!

How do you do that? You know that in that time of need, you need joy so you ask the Father to supply Joy and He will or you can simply turn it on. You decide which way you want to flow in your emotions and in your spirit and this determines the result that you will get. Think about that for a moment.

The Holy Spirit is the spirit of Joy

"For the kingdom of God is not meat and drink; but righteousness, and peace, and joy in the Holy Ghost" - Romans 14:17

The three most potent pillars of the Kingdom of God are listed in this Scripture and they are

1. Righteousness
2. Peace
3. Joy in the Holy Spirit

Righteousness: The Kingdom of God is powered by the force of righteousness. This is what gives birth to the Grace of God and brings us eternal life by Jesus Christ our Lord. Romans 5; 21 Righteousness is what rules the Kingdom of God and this is supplied and credited into our account as we give our lives to Christ, you and I cannot attain to righteousness, we cannot work for it, it is also a gift of God.

This is what governs everything we do, this facilitates our exemption from calamity and destruction. Righteousness is our passage in life, it gives us access to the rich treasury of God, it keeps the enemy in His place, he cannot accuse you, you have been made right with God, He himself has justified you. If the enemy does not have anything on you, he cannot accomplish his mission.

Peace: Everything Thrives in an environment of peace. Any one that promises peace and can remotely give any semblance of it right now will become a god in this present world. Peace is what the world needs more than anything right now, but it can only be found in the Kingdom of God. In our anchor scripture in this book which is Isaiah 53: 4 and 5, one of the key things is that, Jesus took all the punishment and penalty, for our peace and paid the price required to bring us peace. That is how important peace is to God. His plan for you and I is peace Jeremiah 29: 11 He proved that by paying a high price to establish peace for us. Jesus is our Peace. He is the Prince of Peace. He is the price for our peace. He is my peace.

Joy: In an unexpected way, Joy shows up as one of the three core elements of the Kingdom of God to show us the part that Joy plays in our lives. We should have this force of God working in our lives always. It flows from the indwelling presence of the Holy spirit, so we can draw from it as the fountain of life whenever we need to and it will deliver to us that part of our inheritance that we have need in. Healing will come, deliverance and breakthroughs will surely come.

14

God will do for us what He said He will do

Abraham hoped against hope and yet continued to hope. It is said of Him that

Who against hope believed in hope, that he might become the father of many nations, according to that which was spoken, so shall thy seed be. 19 And being not weak in faith, he considered not his own body now dead, when he was about an hundred years old, neither yet the deadness of Sara's womb: 20 He staggered not at the promise of God through unbelief; but was strong in faith, giving glory to God; 21 And being fully persuaded that, what he had promised, he was able also to perform. 22 And therefore it was imputed to him for righteousness. Romans 4: 18 - 22

You do not fight in the day of battle – You rest.

The only fight that we are listed in is the fight of faith, other than that, we are instructed to enter into the rest of faith. Rest can only be borne out of trust, complete trust that the one you have believed is faithful enough to do for you what you have believed Him for. There are a few invitations in the word of God, and one of such invitations is God calling us into the place of rest.

While the enemy will want to get you into worry resulting in doubt and unbelief leading to fear, God said that our only labour should be into that place of rest. This place of rest is where God Himself dwells. God dwells in rest and He said join me in place of my finished work.

When Brother Copeland entered into rest, his healing came. Why is that? Because God is in the place of rest and our peace is in this place, all our supply and provision is in this place of rest. Our healing and sound health is here. Our access into this place is faith and that is why everything and every voice will contend to keep us out of this place.

The supernatural life operates in the place of faith and rest. When we come into this place, we enter into the realm of the Supernatural, which is the realm of God. Mind you this is where your labour is, to do what it takes not to try and be healed or delivered, but to enter the place of faith and rest. When you come into this place, you will find God there and everything you need is in God. this place is where every finished Work manifest.

Again, I say Faith Rests

Brother Kenneth Copeland shared his experience and it has really blessed me. He said he was believing God for healing and he did all that he knew to do to shake it off, but this time it persisted. He decided to get alone and spend time with the Lord and as He did so, he inquired of the Lord why the condition persisted and the Lord said this to him – you are trying too hard – faith rests. He said that took all the pressure off him and when he rests and put that situation in the hand of the Lord, sure enough, his healing came.

Faith Trusts

I heard him say again recently – do not try to make it happen, it has already been accomplished, just receive it and rest. This obviously will only come from a place of trust and absolute persuasion not a halfhearted effort to believe. We must believe in the same way that we believe our Salvation to be true, our healing and health is therefore true also.

**We overcome by the Blood of the Lamb
God will perform His word as we believe**

Testimonies

———◆———

The Scriptures says that the "testimony of Jesus Christ, is the spirit of Prophecy" Revelation 19: 10 Testimonies are prophetic and will reproduce in the life of the one that hears and believes. Testimonies like the word of God produces faith in our hearts and helps us to believe and shows us what to do, because what He does for one He will do for another.

Let this short clip of what is a life changing experience strengthen you to stand in your place of faith knowing that God is faithful who has made the promises to us that we believe and act on.

The Lord said Rest

A servant of God shared that he had symptoms in his body and as usual he began to make declarations of healing scriptures expecting that the symptoms will leave as it always did, but this time it persisted and he began to confess more aggressively in frustration and still nothing happened.

So, he decided to go into his boat alone with God to find out why things are not happening the way that it usually did. He said as he settled down and asked the Lord why, the Lord said to him that he should rest, He said that faith rests and so if he rest, that healing will come, and it did.

What is this saying to us? When we fret and panic in the face of a persisting challenge, we are in essence trying to make it happen and panic brings us out of the place of faith and trust. We said earlier that it is the place of rest that God lives. It is in rest that God moves on our behalf, it is in the place of rest that faith is. Rest is the highest place of faith, it has its foundation in trust that God will not fail, He will do for us what we have trusted Him for simply based on His word.

Quietly trusting

Reverend Bosworth a dynamic early 19th century Evangelist shared this testimony of how that in the face of threatening illness he would often say to the one that he minsters to come into the place of "quietly trusting" he said that was what he did when challenged, he comes into a place of calm assurance – Quietly trusting God to deliver him and bring a turnaround to that situation, sure enough, God always does.

The thought of quietly trusting God to do for you what He has promised which you have received and released your faith for is very re-assuring in the face of contrary circumstance. So, the Word to you today is – "quietly trusting" that God will do for you what He has promised in His word concerning your area of need.

You are healed

Br Kenneth E Hagin shared a testimony of a servant of God that was plagued by Tuberculosis. This servant of God was well known and had a large congregation. Every renowned healing Minister of his day had laid hands on him and prayed the prayer of faith but seemingly he was not healed.

Eventually, he was in the last stages of the disease and he went home to be with his close family to face the obvious. He had a young family and he was kept in a back room by himself because he could hardly move. He said that as he lay there, he decided to exercise his faith in his healing, so he used all the energy he had and left the house into the bushes at the back of the house and literarily dragged himself so far out and collapsed under a tree. He said that the thought had come to him that he has been prayed for and according to the word of God he is now healed.

At this point his mind began to rebuke him for being so stupid to do what he did and now he thought to himself, I will certainly die and no one will find me in the bush because I do not even have the strength to shout enough to be heard by anyone.

So, he decided that, if it is true that he is healed in spite of how he felt, in spite of what the doctors have said, he said, he will lie there and begin to give God the glory for healing him. He began to worship God in that place, forgetting his condition he could barely whisper but he praised God for healing him [remember that is what Abraham, the father of faith and our great example of faith in God did- he did not stagger at the promise of God through unbelieve, but was strong in faith giving Glory to God. Romans 4: 20] and as this preacher kept doing so, strength began to come and his voice was getting louder until he voice was heard so far away. That was his turning point, he began to recover and was completely free.

He decided to believe in spite of the facts before him, he believed anyway that he was healed and so he was.

The word is Medicine

A servant of God also shared her testimony of how she had a lump in her breast, she thought to herself that if things got to the point where she was put in ICU the doctors will put her on hourly round the clock medication, so she began to do as they would do in that situation, she began to take in the Scriptures on healing at the same frequency and the condition cleared up completely.

Dodi Osteen also was diagnosed with cancer and was at the stage where nothing could be done for her though medical science, she had to go home and put her house in order. What she rather did was to collect every Scriptures on healing and then she began to take them as medicine daily.

Her testimony has blessed millions all over the world and her healing book has blessed many. She was totally healed and free and she said that she has not stopped taking her medicine because she was healed, she continues to take her healing Scriptures daily to this day.

The word of God is our Medicine. Proverbs 4: 22 says: "For they are life to those who find them, healing and health to all their flesh" The word of God is living and active, Jesus said "the words that I speak, they are spirit and they are life" The word of God will do exactly what God says. If it speaks of healing, as you receive it into your heart, it will bring healing. The presence of the word that is believed and acted upon will release the power of God into that situation and force a change for you.

Take the Word of God on healing daily alongside your medication if you are on any, soon enough guess which one must bow, the medication will certainly bow out and the word of God will prevail over that condition. The Word of God is your medicine, use it by faith daily.

My Testimony – My heart is fixed trusting the Lord

When I am confronted by a situation, I always run to the word. This has become my way of life. I have no confidence in any other thing but the Word of God. I often say to myself when fear wants to come or when a situation persists that if nothing in this life works for me, the word of God must answer for me. Sure enough it does.

The word of God in my spirit will steadily guide me out of any situation. King David puts it this way and it blesses me. He said in Psalm 56: 3 "What time I am afraid; I will trust in thee. 4 In God I will praise his word, in God I have put my trust" He also said in Psalms 23:4 - "Yea, though I walk through the valley of the shadow of death, I will fear no evil: for thou art with me; thy rod and thy staff they comfort me" The rod and staff here means, the Word and the Spirit. The Holy Spirit and the Word work together to deliver us from any depth of evil and distress. It is the word that I have taken in for many years that will rise to defend me in times of trouble.

Recently instead of having the usual monthly period common to women, but I began to bleed and I expected it to last for a few days as usual but it continued for a period of three weeks, I continued to take in my daily dose of the Word but it persisted so I went to see the Doctor who gave me prescription that it was due to a buildup and that it would clear, but it did not so I became concerned and then my mind began to suggest many things.

At this point my focus was to absolutely keep fear away. I also kept my eye and heart on the word. Even when I was visibly upset, all that came out of my mouth was the Word that I have believed for many years. At some point, Kenneth Copeland shared a testimony about how the Lord gave him the word to stop a situation, that got my attention but I was not expecting it to happen straight away, as I went to the bathroom I heard the Word come out of my spirit "be dry" I immediately knew that I had just been given my word in season, I took that word and began to declare over my womb commanding it to be dry.

It continued but I stayed with the word, I had gone to where that scripture was and found that the Lord also said, "and I will dry up your rivers" meaning that the source of that bleeding will be cut off. So, I kept on declaring that. I went back to the Doctor and I was placed on another medication and the Doctor said something that kept coming to contend with me, he said, it will not stop it, he did not say it may not, he said "it will not stop it" but I had turned around and said to him walking out of that office, I said, it will be alright.

When I got home, I thought maybe I did not respond in faith instantly enough, but I continued to say that over the words of the Doctor, the word of God said, "be dry" so you will dry up. Sure enough at the end of that second set of medication, the bleeding dried up. So, you can work with your Doctor using the medication and the word and the Spirit to accomplish your deliverance. But the key point here is that, we must be filled with the word of God for a day like this one.

With the word working actively inside me, I was calm and trusting, at the point that fear wants to come, I asked the Holy spirit to give me that word that will make me peaceful and restful as He always does. When I experience any challenge and I reach out to God in His word, there is always a word that He will bring that settles things for me and no matter what I am at peace and from then on, the word forces a change.

In this situation, when things persisted, I asked the Holy spirit for that settled word and instantly He gave me – "my heart is fixed trusting the Lord" for there shall no evil befall me" and it is found in Psalm 112, Job 5 and Psalm 91 and Complete rest came and deliverance was established for me. To God alone be all the Glory!

From my heart to your heart

This is the word that the Lord gave to me and I thought I leave that with you. I have found a place in God that I have decided to live in and that place is the place of Mercy. Over and above everything, God's mercy will bring you out of that situation and give you a testimony to the Glory of His name! He said, "For I will be merciful to their unrighteousness, and their sins and their iniquities will I remember no more" Hebrews 8:12

I am saying to you with confidence that "all will surely be well" and you will testify as I have done! Isaiah 12

A call to salvation

If this material has been given to you as a gift and you do not already know Jesus as your Lord and Saviour, now is the perfect opportunity to do so. You see, only as a child of God through salvation in Jesus Christ will you benefit from the terms of this covenant. The scriptures declare;

Neither is there salvation in any other: for there is none other name under heaven given among men, whereby we must be saved. And Romans 10:13 says; "For whosoever shall call upon the name of the Lord shall be saved". Acts 4:12 -

This is how we all get saved by faith

That if thou shalt confess with thy mouth the Lord Jesus, and shalt believe in thine heart that God hath raised him from the dead, thou shalt be saved.

10 For with the heart man believeth unto righteousness; and with the mouth confession is made unto salvation. Romans 10:9.

Pray this prayer and believe.

Father I confess with my mouth That Jesus Christ is Lord and I believe in my heart that you raised Him from the dead. Lord Jesus I open my heart to you, come into my heart and become my Lord and Saviour, forgive all my sin and accept me now into your kingdom, Lord fill me with your Holy Spirit. I receive salvation now and I am filled with the Holy Spirit in Jesus name, amen.

It does not stop there, after we receive Jesus as our Lord and Saviour, we get into fellowship with the brethren, so ask the Lord to lead you to the right place of fellowship and especially get a good Bible and Christian books and messages to build your faith as we have heard in this material to enable your growth and spiritual understanding.

Finally, I commit you to God and to the Holy Spirit, as it is written: "And now, brethren, I commend you to God, and to the word of his grace, which is able to build you up, and to give you an inheritance among all them which are sanctified". Acts20: 32. Be Blessed!

About Heavenly Life Ministries

We are a ministry in response to the instruction of our Lord Jesus Christ in;

"All power is given unto me in heaven and in earth. 19 Go ye therefore, and teach all nations, baptizing them in the name of the Father, and of the Son, and of the Holy Ghost: 20 teaching them to observe all things whatsoever I have commanded you: and, lo, I am with you always, even unto the end of the world. Amen." Mat 28: 18 - 20

Go ye into all the world, and preach the gospel to every creature. 16 He that believeth and is baptized shall be saved; but he that believeth not shall be damned. 17 And these signs shall follow them that believe; in my name shall they cast out devils; they shall speak with new tongues; 18 they shall take up serpents; and if they drink any deadly thing, it shall not hurt them; they shall lay hands on the sick, and they shall recover.

So then after the Lord had spoken unto them, he was received up into heaven, and sat on the right hand of God. 20 And they went forth, and preached everywhere The Lord working with them and confirming the word with signs following Amen Mark 16: 15 – 21

We do exactly this through the following platform:
- The Working Document Books
- Media and Publications
-The feed my Lamb Project/Foundation
Education. Scholarships – Small Business Finance and Training Programs
- Weekly and monthly Community wide distribution of Gospel Tracts and Bibles

Our true Heritage in Christ Jesus can only be found in the Word of God, as it is written: "And now, brethren, I commend you to God, and to the word of his grace, which is able to build you up, and to give you an inheritance among all them which are sanctified. Acts 20:32

ABOUT THE AUTHOR

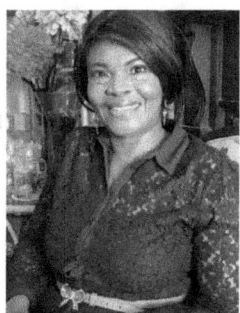

Margaret Ema is an Author and Speaker and co-director in Heavenly Life Ministries worldwide. BSc Hons in Digital Technology Innovation and creativity and holds a Post graduate certificate in International Management Liverpool University United Kingdom.

Her focus is Mentorship

She is blessed with 4 Boys and God's Blessing added Five beautiful daughters.

Other Titles from this Author include

- Holy Spirit – The Healer Within You
- Faith in God – Power to do the Impossible
- Faith – Let Jesus show you how to use your faith on Purpose
- God inside you – Unlimited Capacity
- We Live in Light – Understanding Your advantage
- Amazing Blessing
- Let there be – and it is so – and it is Good
- Morning Glory – Your daily Building Material
- Health and Cure – Do you know your Rights in God?
- Health and Cure – Quick read
- Like God – Living now in the Realm of GOD
- You must fear no evil!
- Marriage is a Blessing
- Marriage: Enjoyment not Endurance
- Just Married – Naked and not ashamed
- Use your Faith – Your Life Depends on it

Contact us: connect@heavenlylife.org

Notes

Notes

Notes

Notes